WEIGHT LOSS
STARTS IN YOUR BRAIN™

The CogniDiet®

The Companion Book

100 **(Almost)** Experiments to **Rewire** Your Brain, **Lose** the Weight and **Enjoy** Life!

The CogniDiet®
Weight Loss Starts in Your Brain
The Companion Book

Published by
The CogniDiet
Princeton, NJ
www.TheCogniDiet.com

ISBN: 978-0-578-41977-0
Printed in the United States
Cover design and layout by 20 Lemons, LLC

Table of Contents

The Final Four Weeks: The Master Level

You Are a Master!

Introduction

I am so excited to be back with this new book, a companion to my 2018 book, *Weight Loss Starts in Your Brain*. After working with this program, many of my clients and readers asked for a companion book mixing games and experiments to help readers adopt new behaviors and grow in confidence each week as the experiments become more challenging.

For example, instead of only reading the chapter "How to Deal with Emotional Eating," now there are 12 specific "emotional eating" experiments, one per week, in this new book. Each week you will learn and experience something new and be able to move on to the next. Each week the pounds will be shed forever! That is the goal.

You can choose to follow only one of the seven transformational themes developed in my CogniDiet® Program to lose weight. This is a holistic experience merging the heart, mind, and body. Weight loss can only occur if you take care of these seven elements, which conveniently mirror the seven days of the week:

 1. NUTRITION IQ AND FOOD EXPERIENCES

2. ACTIVITY LEVEL AND ENERGY

3. EMOTIONS

4. SELF-LOVE

5. MINDFULNESS AND ZEN LIFE

6. DEALING WITH STRESS

7. LIFE HACKS TO SIMPLIFY YOUR LIFE

Seven Experiments per Week – Three Levels of Mastery

The book is organized in three sections representing increasing levels of mastery. Each section is four weeks long. Each week the experiments become more challenging in level of self-control and behavioral mastery. This book is designed for you to follow over 12 weeks, so enjoy the journey and take it at a slow pace.

Certain skills must be learned before you can advance to the next level. This book is not about teaching you something specific, as my first book was. Instead, it will help you "change by doing." I highly recommend you read *Weight Loss Starts in Your Brain* prior to working with the experiments in this book in order to understand the reasoning behind the experiments, including cutting sugar, eating unsaturated fat, or tackling your emotions.

This book does not go into explaining the science behind a game and will only include a brief rationale.

The first four weeks are the Beginner Level. Do not skip this part of the journey, even if you are already familiar with The CogniDiet® techniques and principles. It is always good to go back to the basics.

When you have achieved this level at the end of the first four weeks, you move to the Advanced Level for another four weeks. After these four weeks, you will be ready to advance to the Mastery Level.

You may be slower than others at losing weight, you may be less disciplined or have a more complicated or challenging life. It is okay. Everyone should go at their own pace.

Here are a few ways to advance through the weeks:
- Follow the weeks and experiments as advised, one each day.
- Go at a slower pace and take, for instance, two or more weeks if needed, to cover all seven experiments of a specific week.
- Only follow one theme at a time and focus, for example, on just "self-love" or "mindfulness" for 12 weeks.
- Redo a week's curriculum if you feel you did not master it.
- Return to previous weeks' experiments to see the progress you made on past challenges.
- Repeat experiments if necessary, as many times as you want. This is very important because it may require a few times to really bear the fruits of new learning.

Here are a few things to do to be successful in this exciting endeavor:
- Create and write down your goals.
- Create your vision board and make it visible—see Chapter 1 in *Weight Loss Starts in Your Brain*.
- Measure progress and be accountable to yourself.
- Decide on a nutrition and exercise/activity plan before you start.
- Encourage friends and family to do the experiments in this book with you. Why not? You can compare results and support each other.
- Know your baseline data—more to come on this.
- Note your findings and observations in this book, or another booklet.
- Have faith in yourself.

Build Your Goals

Here are a few tips to build SMART goals:

S is for **Specific**: Be clear on what you want to achieve from a weight, fat to muscle ratio, or even health-related issue such as lowering your blood pressure or A1C. Start by having a physical and getting baseline numbers for lipids panel, glucose, blood pressure, and liver panel. Repeat these tests at the end of the journey.

M is for **Measurable**: Be accountable and have a defined goal for each week.

A is for **Achievable**: Do not say you plan to lose 40 pounds in 12 weeks if you have not been able to lose 10 pounds in the last 10 years; a half to two pounds a week is a great success; sustainable weight loss must be slow. Be ambitious, but also reasonable.

R is for **Relevant or Realistic**: Try to align your goals with your lifestyle. Do not say you want to run a marathon in a year if you know life will really get in the way of the time needed to train. Instead commit to three 10K races in a year.

T is for **Time-Oriented**: I have noticed over the years that people are very ambitious in terms of achievements, and also impatient. Saying you want to lose 10 pounds is not enough. You have to write "I will lose 10 pounds before the end of September."

Cogni-Tips for the Road

- Try to be as organized and as committed as you can to the program. You can decide to follow it for only six weeks, but whatever you decide, do it.

- If you do it, do it well—even if you skip a week. Go back and keep at it. Sometimes you may need to repeat a week because you struggled.

- Try to schedule your training sessions and food plan in advance.

- Measure your success weekly, or even daily if that makes you feel better. Celebrate often!

- Do the experiments with a friend and encourage each other. Share your experiment results. Create a club such as the book club recommended in *Weight Loss Starts in Your Brain*.

- Write down every success or setback you achieve. Writing things down is part of the brain rewiring methodology.

- Reward yourself.

You will learn and change by doing and reflecting on each experience. You will also build up your confidence while you rewire your brain. This is a self-discovery journey.

Let's start with writing what are your goals, commitment level, and self-motivating motto for the next 12 weeks.

Write your SMART weight loss and life goals:

_____

_____

_____

_____

Write your self-motivating motto:

_____

_____

Create a food and drink elimination list:

_____

_____

_____

Create a new healthy food discovery list:

_____

_____

_____

_____

Write the list of behaviors and other things you want to really change:

_____

_____

_____

List your initial fasting glucose, hemoglobin A1C, and lipid panel (LDL, HDL, triglycerides), and liver data if available:

		INITIAL	WEEK 12
FASTING GLUCOSE			
HEMOGLOBIN A1C			
LIPID PANEL	LDL		
	HDL		
	TRIGLYCERIDES		
LIVER DATA	ALT		
	AST		

Initial Measures

	INITIAL	4 WEEKS	8 WEEKS	FINAL
WEIGHT				
BODY FAT RATIO (if you have a special scale)				
BMI (if available)				
CHEST				
RIGHT UPPER ARM				
LEFT UPPER ARM				
WAIST				
HIPS				
WAIST/HIPS RATIO				
RIGHT THIGH				
LEFT THIGH				
RIGHT CALF				
LEFT CALF				

Let's Start

THE FIRST FOUR WEEKS

The Beginner Level

Week 1

Take Your Baseline Pictures!

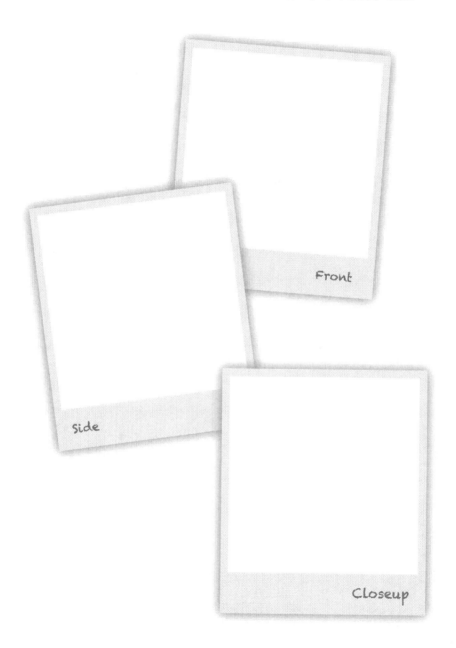

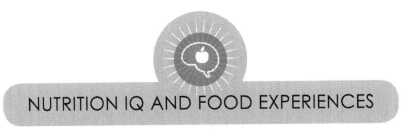

NUTRITION IQ AND FOOD EXPERIENCES

Experiment #1 – Build Sugar Mountains

Read the label on a bag of chips, candy, cookies, or your favorite processed junk processed food. This week eliminate at least one processed snack and replace it with a healthier version or, even better, nothing.

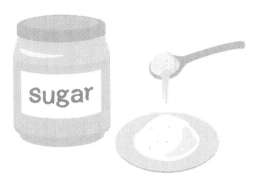

Look at:
- The total calories in the bag (count all servings).
- The number of bites or the portion you typically eat at one sitting. Calculate how many calories this represents.
- The time it took you to eat what you wanted to eat.
- Count all the carbohydrates grams minus fiber and translate this into grams of sugar. **Count one gram of net carbohydrate as one gram of sugar.** If there are 21g of net carbohydrates in the bag, this is 21g of sugar. There are 4g of sugar in a teaspoon, translate this into how many teaspoons of sugar are in front of you. Take out a bag of sugar and put the number of teaspoons of sugar on a plate or your counter.
- Read the label for other information. Look at the list of ingredients. What kind of fat and sugar sources are there? What type of preservatives or food enhancers are listed?

Yes, carbohydrates are also flour and fruits and vegetables, but all carbohydrates, with the exception of fiber, turn into glucose in your blood.

Draw the heaps of sugar representing the net grams of carbohydrates on the bag and note how many teaspoons this represents. If you eat different snacks, continue to add heaps of sugar to the bag.

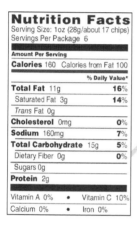

Nutrition Facts
Serving Size: 1oz (28g/about 17 chips)
Servings Per Package 6

Amount Per Serving

Calories 160   Calories from Fat 100

	% Daily Value*
Total Fat 11g	**16%**
Saturated Fat 3g	**14%**
Trans Fat 0g	
Cholesterol 0mg	**0%**
Sodium 160mg	**7%**
Total Carbohydrate 15g	**5%**
Dietary Fiber 0g	**0%**
Sugars 0g	
Protein 2g	

Vitamin A 0%	•	Vitamin C 10%
Calcium 0%	•	Iron 0%

Example
If I eat **half this bag** of chips:
15g of carbs x 3 = 45g.
No fiber, so that's 45g of sugar divided by four – that's over 11 teaspoons of sugar!
AND 160 x 3 = 480 calories!

What did you learn?

_____

_____

_____

Rationale and benefits of this experiment:
The goal is to make you realize how many calories, preservatives, net carbohydrates, and sugar you ingest when you eat processed snacks.

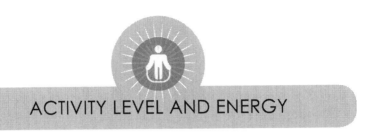

ACTIVITY LEVEL AND ENERGY

Experiment #2 – Let's Push It!

Today make one decision about your activity and exercise regimen. It is time to go to the next level. Rest assured, we will take your current fitness level into account.

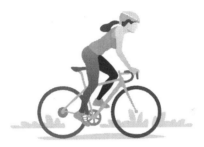

Are you a beginner, intermediate, or a professional exerciser?

Beginners = Almost zero exercise.
Do at least one of these three things:

- Start walking 20 minutes a day at a brisk pace. Walk around your neighborhood every morning or evening. Find a walking buddy.
- Sign up and go to the gym at least once a week.
- Buy a pedometer to see how many steps you walk each day. If you realize you were not exceeding 2,000 to 5,000 steps a day, each week add 1,000 to 2,000 steps a day, until you regularly log in 10,000 to 12,000 steps a day. You can use an average for the week.

Intermediate = You exercise, but only once or twice a week, or you are not pushing yourself.
Do at least one of these three things:

- Add steps every day in 1,000 increments.

- Add one more day at the gym to at least twice a week or add another weekly activity to make you move and sweat.
- Try a new class if you feel bored.

Professional = You are very committed and disciplined, but you can't seem to lose the weight.
Do at least one of these three things:
- Have you fallen into a rut: same elliptical, same pace, same classes? Try something new.
- Increase intensity either in number of reps, heart rate, time, etc.
- Try a new sport or activity.
- Embark on a fitness evaluation with a professional and take stock of what needs to be improved.

Write your plan NOW and don't forget to think about all aspects of training your body:

GOALS	PAST	AS OF TODAY, AND FOR THE NEXT 12 WEEKS
CARDIO		
STRENGTH TRAINING		
FLEXIBILITY/ RELAXATION (for example, yoga)		
WALKING		

Rationale and benefits of this experiment:
By boosting your current level, you may get out of a routine not allowing you to really burn calories effectively. If you are a couch potato, now is time to start moving!

EMOTIONS

Experiment #3 – I Know My Emotions

Are you emotional? When feeling an emotion, or in order not to feel it, do you turn to food? Are you dealing with anger or sadness with a cookie or ice cream?

Even happy emotions, such as joy, can trigger a craving as a kind of reward or association. Do you say to yourself, "Because I succeeded and got an A+ on this exam, I deserve a reward?"

Let's face it. Some of us always find reasons for reward. A lot of us do not recognize the underlying emotions acting as triggers for a candy frenzy. Before embarking on dealing with emotional eating you must first have the courage to face and understand your underlying emotions.

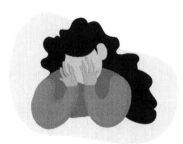

This week is the first step. This week, if and when you feel an emotion coming, note how you feel. Write down your words to describe it in this book or in a booklet.

Do not judge yourself. Do not feel guilty. Be kind to yourself. Only note the emotion(s). Then note what happens after you ate that cookie or treat.

DAY	EMOTION(S)	HOW DO YOU FEEL AFTER YOU'VE HAD A TREAT?
DAY 1		
DAY 2		
DAY 3		
DAY 4		
DAY 5		
DAY 6		
DAY 7		

Rationale and benefits of this experiment:

You will become more self-aware of your emotions and their triggers. You will begin to see patterns. You will understand what the "treat" does to you. Does it solve your underlying emotion?

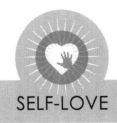

SELF-LOVE

Experiment #4 – My Best Assets

Loving yourself is so crucial. If you love yourself, you become gentler with yourself, and committed to your own well-being. You do not punish yourself, you treat yourself with respect and consideration.

This week write five physical traits you love about yourself, such as your eyes, your feet, your hair, or your legs. Whatever. They are your best assets, the ones you flaunt easily because they give you confidence. Today you will be more specific about why you love them.

A few examples of what to write:

- I love my eyes because they have an amazingly clear blue color and long lashes.
- I love my skin because it is so soft, and it has a nice caramel color.
- I love my legs because they are long, well defined, and muscular.

Rationale and benefits of this experiment:
Loving yourself is the first step towards feeling good. The better you feel, the easier it is to shed pounds because you will be focused on the positive rather than the negative aspects of your body.

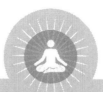

MINDFULNESS AND ZEN LIFE

Experiment #5 – I Am Out for Lunch!

Enjoy life. Become more mindful of the
moment, be in the moment, and go with the
flow. Don't be on your smart phone while
having lunch with your family. Don't manage
your Instagram account while walking in the
woods. You can post these pictures later!

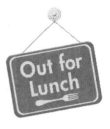

Today at lunch or dinner—or choose another day this week if
you are too busy professionally—plan to sit down at meal time,
with no distraction and for at least 15 to 20 minutes eat on your
own.

Enjoy the view, the textures, and the flavors. Think about where
this food is coming from. Chew slowly and be thankful for this
delicious meal. You can do this at home or in the office at your
desk, but it is forbidden to work!

After the meal, write how you feel. Start with "I feel" or
"I am," etc.

Rationale and benefits of this experiment:
*You may notice you eat less when you eat slowly
because you become satisfied quicker. You are also
immersed in the action. This may lower your cravings
later. It decreases your stress level because eating will
have been an enjoyable moment and not something
on your "To Do" list.*

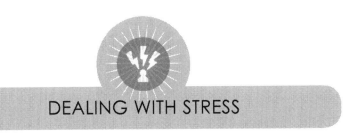

DEALING WITH STRESS

Experiment #6 – I Know When I'm Stressed

Do you even know how stressed you are? We multitask, and juggle commitments and we run on adrenaline all day.

The first step in starting to better manage stress is to be aware of it and notice your level. Using the *Weight Loss Starts in Your Brain* book scale:

0 (none, never)   **5** (reasonably)   **10** (huge, all the time)

Take the day and regularly measure the level of stress you feel. Notice the patterns, the way you feel, and the culprits. You can compare days of the week. Do this a few days this week.

DAY OF WEEK: _____

Morning: _____

Afternoon: _____

Evening: _____

Notes: _____

DAY OF WEEK: _____

Morning: _____

Afternoon: _____

Evening: _____

Notes: _____

DAY OF WEEK: _____

Morning: _____

Afternoon: _____

Evening: _____

Notes: _____

DAY OF WEEK: _____

Morning: _____

Afternoon: _____

Evening: _____

Notes: _____

What have you noticed? What are you learning about yourself?
Notice your body feelings (hands shaking, cravings, not
breathing properly, lack of focus, feeling lost, etc.).

Rationale and benefits of this experiment:
*You become aware of how long and how seriously you
have been stressed, and what the causes of your stress
are. This is the first step to start dealing with it.*

LIFE HACKS TO SIMPLIFY YOUR LIFE

Experiment #7 – Carry Your Own Food

Simplify your life by planning. It does not take much time, and it allows for more free time and control later. One thing I noticed over the years is that people struggling with weight loss are at the mercy of events or situations. They may use this as an excuse, but if you plan your day, as much as you can, there are no excuses left.

This week, plan your meals for the next three days. I am only asking three days to start with! A few tips:

- Cook the night before and bring leftovers to work the next day.
- Cook meals that last two or three days, such as casseroles, whole chicken, etc.
- Cook batches of vegetables and soups and freeze in single serving portions.
- If you can control yourself, have healthy snacks at your disposal at the office, in your car, or bag.

A few ideas for this week:

_____

_____

_____

Rationale and benefits of this experiment:
You will have more control on your environment and stop succumbing to bad cafeteria food or the snack machine.

Week 2

We hope you had a great first week. If you already amped up the calorie cut and energy burning factors, you should start seeing results. Was it hard? If you struggled, regroup, and repeat the Week 1 curriculum without guilt.

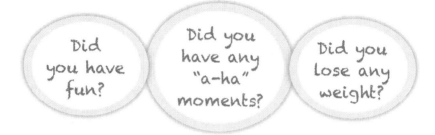

Did you have fun?

Did you have any "a-ha" moments?

Did you lose any weight?

Reread some of the chapters in *Weight Loss Starts in Your Brain*. It will give you the foundational knowledge of the science behind certain foods—remember sugar is not your friend—and some experiments.

As you start Week 2, draw something that captures how you feel. As I am writing, I feel like a flying squirrel!

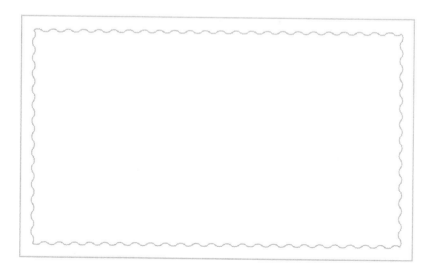

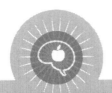

NUTRITION IQ AND FOOD EXPERIENCES

Experiment #8 – Snack Eliminator

This week eliminate something you know is sabotaging your efforts. Is it the nightly pretzel snack, the afternoon 500 calorie ice cream, the three times a week large pizza slice? Whatever it is, eliminate it or make a healthy swap. For example:

- 10 nuts (80 to 120 calories) instead of a bag of chips or pretzels.
- A 100-150 calorie yogurt versus a serving of ice cream.
- Pizza once a week versus three times a week.
- One glass of wine versus two a night.

Make your resolution and commit to it NOW: This week I will eliminate or change:

_____

_____

_____

Cogni-Tip: You can eliminate more than one thing, but don't deprive yourself of every one of your little pleasures at once.

Rationale and benefits of this experiment:
This will accelerate your weight loss and after one week allow you to see you can live without one of these snacks or foods you were so attached to. It may help you cut 2,000 to 3,000 calories a week.

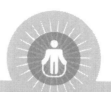

ACTIVITY LEVEL AND ENERGY

Experiment #9 – I Know My Data

You started to accelerate and strengthen your activity level. And hopefully it works. So please, continue. This week be courageous and know your numbers. Not everybody will have the desire or discipline to take all the body measurements I asked you to take in the introduction (go to page 7, if not done yet). I want you to know your percentage of body fat. A healthy one is around 30-35% for the average sized woman and 25-30% for the average sized man. There are tables available online for you to check. They take into consideration gender, age, and physical condition.

Are you classified as healthy, overweight, obese, or extremely obese? Traditional home scales only tell one part of the story. Newer scales now measure body fat (not totally reliable but at least they will give you a baseline), or you can ask at your gym or the doctor's office to be measured. Worst case scenario, you can use your Body Mass Index (BMI) which is not ideal but will give you an indication. Tables are also available online.

My percent of body fat and/or BMI is: _____

My goal is to lower it to: _____

Rationale and benefits of this experiment:
It is easy to ignore numbers and/or rationalize them by ethnic, morphological, or genetic considerations. If you are classified as obese or extremely obese, face reality, but be reasonable. It takes time to change a body.

Remember: Continue to exercise this week…

Experiment #10 – My Top Emotions

Last week you started to find out and put a name to the emotions behind your cravings. This week make a list of the top three to five emotions that come up most of the time before a craving occurs.

 Cogni-Tip: Stress-related cravings are not emotionally based cravings. Boredom is also not an emotion. Let's stay focused on the real emotions.

The emotion can be joy, sadness, envy, jealousy, loneliness, happiness, etc. It can be positive or negative.

My top three to five emotions are _____

_____

_____

The next time it occurs explain WHY you feel this emotion. For example, "I feel angry because my daughter did not call me." Ask yourself, "Why am I angry?" Write it down and reflect upon it, instead of immediately going for ice cream.

My emotion was _____

I am _____ because

_____

_____

_____

 Rationale and benefits of this experiment:
You will start to peel off, understand, and face your emotions, instead of ignoring them with a piece of candy, which is a form of distraction. It is not easy, but you can tackle one emotion at a time.

Remember: You may benefit from seeing a psychotherapist if you feel the emotions are deeply set and require professional help.

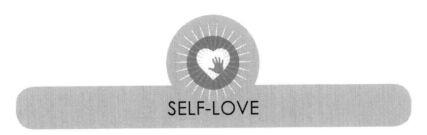

SELF-LOVE

Experiment #11 – My Numerous Talents

This week, make a list of talents, skills, and positive personality traits you possess. Ask family or friends for help, especially if you are modest or lack self-confidence. Write them down and then think about how you can leverage them for this journey.

A few examples of what to write: "I am very well-organized at home and at the office, so I can use this skill to become better at planning my meals." "I am a gifted painter and artist. Next time I feel a craving coming, I should doodle something to express how I feel instead of reaching for a chocolate."

Write down your top skills and talents. Express them starting with the word "I." Focus on the top five:

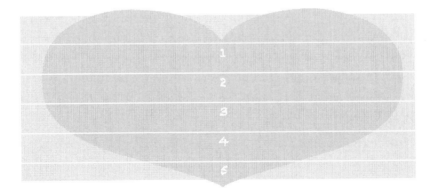

1

2

3

4

5

Rationale and benefits of this experiment:
This will help you build confidence and focus on what will help you succeed, rather than what will make you fail. It will also give you a higher success rate.

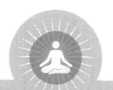

MINDFULNESS AND ZEN LIFE

Experiment #12 – Make a Movie in Your Head!

Today find a moment to take a 10-minute break wherever you are, no excuses. Take a walk or sit still and alone at your desk or somewhere.

 Cogni-Tip: Getting in your car is a good way to have alone time. Just be on your own.

During this break you absolutely must avoid messaging, calling, or any distraction such as eating or drinking. Put your phone on silent, or, even better, don't take it with you. Friends, family, and colleagues can live without you for 10 minutes.

Close your eyes. Breathe gently through your nostrils. Be seated comfortably. Let go of any negative energy or tension in your body. Think about a nice memory, picture this as vividly as you can, create a mini story in your head as if this memory was a movie. You are the director. Picture something that really happened and made you happy and fulfilled.

How do you feel after? Write it down immediately.

I feel _____

_____

_____

_____

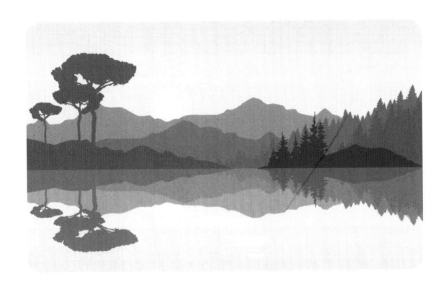

Rationale and benefits of this experiment:

It will calm your brain and distract you from stress. Conjuring happy moments is called visualization and promotes calmness. You may avoid a craving because your brain received a serotonin boost, which increases a feeling of happiness, via something other than a snack. Repeat every time you feel down, stressed, sad, or are on the path to experiencing another food bingeing episode.

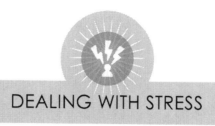

DEALING WITH STRESS

Experiment #13 – How Bad Is It?

You are starting to realize what triggers your stress – and it is not emotions. This is different. What stresses you out are SITUATIONS or PEOPLE (who create situations). This week continue to observe your level of stress but start to relativize it.

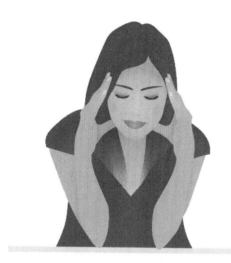

Answer these questions:

1. *Is this situation life endangering?*
   This includes death, serious disease, bankruptcy, or job loss. Will it change your life? Or did you just miss a train, get stuck in traffic, or miss a deadline, which are all fixable problems.

2. *Is this under my control?*

Maybe you could have paid your credit card on time and avoided penalties, but you did not. You decided to pay it late. If you are bad at managing your budget, enroll in a financial literacy class and/or negotiate a better interest-bearing card or speak with your bank. MOST PROBLEMS ARE UNDER YOUR CONTROL. What problems are not under your control? Earthquakes, floods, a major health emergency, or accidents involving yourself or a loved one.

Relativize the source of stress. People today stress over holiday season shopping, wedding planning, vacations, family dinners… MUST YOU?

Action: Take a deep breath and face your stress sources. Choose one major source of stress. Either minimize, eliminate, or consider a long-term plan to deal with it.

Rationale and benefits of this experiment:
This will teach you to relativize your stress level. You must learn not to stress about what you cannot control and what is relatively minor.

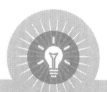

LIFE HACKS TO SIMPLIFY YOUR LIFE

Experiment #14 – Focus Please!

Nowadays we run around like chickens with our heads cut off because DOING is what makes us feel real and relevant. But how much of what we do each day does not support our goals?

Remember the goals you wrote two weeks ago. Reread them and write what needs to happen to achieve them in one column. In the next column write what needs to disappear in order to achieve them.

NEEDS TO HAPPEN	NEEDS TO BE ELIMINATED

Is eating out four times a week with friends really what you need so you can say you have no time to cook healthy foods? Or is now really the time to start pottery classes (unless it calms you down)? Are you serious about losing weight? It will not happen miraculously. How focused are you?

This is big decision week. Eliminate what is standing in your way.

Rationale and benefits of this experiment:
This exercise will help you FOCUS on what matters in this journey.

Week 3

We have been together now for 14 days. How much weight have you lost?

I have lost _____ pounds.

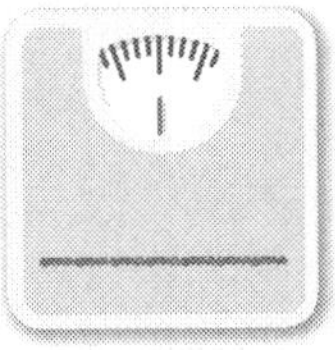

How do you feel overall? Use only a few words.

I feel _____

Have you had a few "a-ha" moments these past two weeks regarding stressors, emotions, and commitment to this journey?

I realized _____

_____

How confident are you that you are changing or will change?

I am _____

What do you want to achieve this week?

I want to _____

_____

Write a word to describe yourself today here!

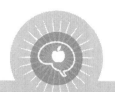

NUTRITION IQ AND FOOD EXPERIENCES

Experiment #15 – Draw Your Plate

Look at what you have eaten in the past few days and visualize this on a plate. How big is your vegetable portion? How large or high is the pasta, fries, or rice portion?

Aim to abide by the 50% vegetables rule. All vegetables are encouraged on that half, except peas, carrots, beets, corn, and potatoes because these are highest in sugar and starch and should be counted as your starch.

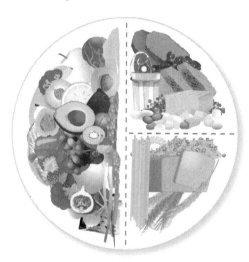

Rationale and benefits of this experiment:
Vegetables are filling, a good source of carbohydrates, anti-oxidants, fiber, and vitamins. Our plates often contain too many starchy carbohydrates, which can trigger future sugar cravings.

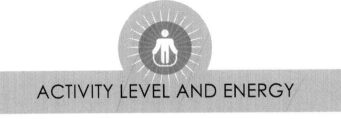

ACTIVITY LEVEL AND ENERGY

Experiment #16 – My Sabotaging Thoughts

This week you also need to self-motivate, especially if you feel frustrated, or a little bit lazy. You know you need to move in order to lose and maintain a healthy weight.

Write a list of all the excuses you use to not exercise, and transform them into positive, life transforming statements (remember the Sabotaging Automatic Thoughts – SATs – versus The Positive Amazing Thoughts – PATs – in Chapter 3 of *Weight Loss Starts in Your Brain*).

For Example: "I am too tired to go to the gym tonight" replace with: "I will feel so much better and re-energized when I come back. I can always only do 30 minutes tonight."

SATs	PATs

SATs	PATs

Rationale and benefits of this experiment:
You rewire your brain with positive thinking, and action and create new, healthier pathways. Think about strategies such as having a gym bag in your car so no excuses are left.

EMOTIONS

Experiment #17 – I Feel the Emotions

How are you doing emotionally? Are you becoming more aware of your feelings? I hope so. In the past, frustration and a feeling of lack of control or failure (lack of self-worth) led me to cupcakes. Now I write an action plan and go for a run instead of heading for the cupcakes. I am asking you to write about the next time an emotion hits you. Observe it without judgment, guilt, or fear. Consider this a science project.

What are your physical feelings? Where does your body hurt? Observe what happens with your breathing, your hands, your general posture, your heart beat, etc. How do you think you look? I know it is hard to describe, but very often an emotion can affect your body in different places, and in different ways.

Write down the whole experience. Focus on physical feelings.

I feel _____

_____

_____

Rationale and benefits of this experiment:
Observing an emotion can help you to let it pass, rather than to resist it. It will also help you realize its seriousness level. You may need the help of a health care practitioner. Stop avoiding resolution.

SELF-LOVE

Experiment #18 – A Treat to Myself

Today reward yourself with a new experience, do something that makes you happy. It can be shared with somebody. It must have to do with something you love about yourself and that you want to celebrate. It could be a coffee with a friend you have not seen in a while, a theater ticket, or even a walk in the city. This is not a material acquisition.

The idea is to gift yourself. After the experience, reflect upon how much something little can make you happy and change the entire flavor of your day. Enjoy the experience to the fullest.

Today I treated myself to _____

_____

It made me feel _____

_____

_____

Rationale and benefits of this experiment:
By doing this you reinforce a happy pathway in your brain. The more you do this, the stronger the pathway becomes. When you are happy, you usually don't think about eating! Make sure you create an emotional memory.

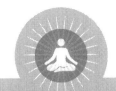

MINDFULNESS AND ZEN LIFE

Experiment #19 – I Take a Forest Bath

Get closer to nature this week. Leave the crowds, the noise, and consumerism. Go to a forest and sit or lie down on a large rock, a fallen tree, or the ground. It is called a "forest bath." You will pick up the earth's energy through this and become one with the trees, the foliage, the earth, and the animals. Perhaps there is a little river humming by. You can decide whether to close your eyes or to simply observe. Do this for at least 30 minutes.

This can be done on a beach, on a boat, or in a hammock in your garden. If you practice meditation, you can simply meditate. You just need to be surrounded by nature and must avoid crowded and noisy places. As you do this, you will not be drinking a sugary treat at a coffee shop. You will not be shopping at a mall. You will not be online. You will be doing something you may not have done before. If you do not want to sit or lie down, then walk. Be on your own. That is the only condition.

How do you feel when you come back?

I feel _____

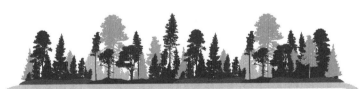

Rationale and benefits of this experiment:
It is well known being in nature has a calming effect on our body and mind.

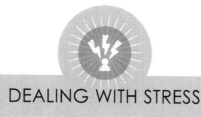

DEALING WITH STRESS

Experiment #20 – Are You Still Breathing?

Let's focus on breathing. Breathing counteracts the stress attack on your body and mind by working on your parasympathetic system – the part of the nervous system that calms you down. It lowers your cortisol level. When we are stressed out, we usually forget to breathe correctly. By breathing deeply, you give extra oxygen to your brain. This is badly needed to continue to function while dealing with an emergency! Always remember to breathe with your whole lungs, and not just the upper part.

Here are a few easy techniques to use for a few minutes the next time you start to feel overwhelmed. Even five minutes can be sufficient. And you can do this discreetly:

1. Count to four and inhale.
2. Hold for four counts.
3. Exhale for four counts.

Repeat a few times. There are other techniques, but in the end, make sure your lungs are completely filled up. Put your hand(s) discreetly on your abdomen and feel them go up and down.

Rationale and benefits of this experiment:
This will calm you down and reground you in your body. It is the cheapest and most under-utilized calming technique! Teach it to your kids, too. You can do this anytime, anywhere.

LIFE HACKS TO SIMPLIFY YOUR LIFE

Experiment #21 – Ditch the Smart Phone

Let's continue to simplify your life. Are you still sure you want to transform your body and mind to achieve a healthier version of YOU?

Scream it: YESSSSSSSSSSSSSSSSSSS!

Today I am asking you to do something really tough. Can you spend less time on social media, Google, and reading the news? Be honest, how many minutes or hours do you spend on social media? A recent study shows we spend an average of two hours and 51 minutes a day (2017 Cross Platform in Focus Report) on our smart phones!

Once you know your score/time (enter here_____), are you surprised or at least feeling a little bit guilty? What are you really getting from this time?

I see people on the phone on the elliptical at the gym and walking in the streets. We see families at the restaurant on their phones, each isolated in their own bubbles. This addiction is taking your life away and keeps you in a dependence mode versus being IN CONTROL of your time.

Once you know how much time you are wasting, write down how many times you plan to check your smart phone in the future. Give yourself a time budget.

Rationale and benefits of this experiment:
Stop complaining you don't have enough time. Be in charge of your life.

Week 4

Last week we asked you to become a little bit more Zen and introspective. We wanted you to get more aligned with your true self.

We hope you were kind, loving and gentle with yourself. Do you feel calmer? We hope so.

What is your level of calmness right now?

☐	Very calm
☐	Somewhat calm
☐	Not at all calm
☐	Will get better in a few minutes

What is your resolution for this week regarding your Zen Factor? Write it down:

_____

_____

_____

 Cogni-Tip: By checking your Zen factor regularly you become calmer and more grounded. You have the tools to make it happen. Calmer = less cravings!

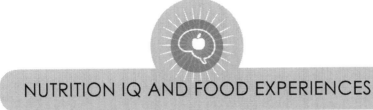

NUTRITION IQ AND FOOD EXPERIENCES

Experiment #22 – The Hunger Game

Gauge your hunger level this week. It is important especially as you start to eat on a smaller plate.

When you are ready to eat, or eating outside of regular meals, measure your hunger level. It is in the *Weight Loss Starts in Your Brain* book, Chapter 7, "I Deal with Saboteurs and Eat Mindfully."

Level 1 is being "famished," Level 5 is being "satisfied or neutral," and Level 10 is being "stuffed!"

This week, before each food encounter, note your hunger level. If it is a Level 5, there is NO reason to eat. And when at Level 6, being satisfied, you should stop eating.

Ask yourself that question:
"If I am not hungry, why would I want to eat this?" It means something else, whether it is emotions, stress, or older habits are driving your hand.

If it is not hunger, it is mindless eating. Repeat this several times.

Rationale and benefits of this experiment:
This is the most important experiment of this entire journey. Eating is not a hobby. Eating is something you do to fuel your body and mind. You must be aware of your hunger level at all times. We are disconnected from it.

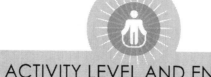

ACTIVITY LEVEL AND ENERGY

Experiment #23 – The 10% Rule

You have been active now for almost four weeks if you are following this program! You are on a path to change. You should see results not only on the scale, but also in your body shape and contouring.

You created your positive affirmations last week. Writing them is one thing. Putting them into action is another. This week mark your exercise or activity level in your weekly planner. Increase your activity level.

Action #1: Increase your activity by 10%. As an example, if you walk two miles a day, now walk 2.2 miles. If you run 30 minutes, add three minutes. If you do 12 reps of a strength routine, do 13. There is nothing preventing you from increasing by 30%, or from going to the gym three times a week versus two times.

Action #2: Write how you feel. After all you are moving more!

Action #1:	I am:
Action #2:	I feel:

Rationale and benefits of this experiment:
Increasing your daily activity by 10% seems minor, but it helps you burn more calories. And writing how you feel after you took the action helps you measure progress, feel encouraged and motivated to continue to step up.

EMOTIONS

Experiment #24 – A Mindful Treat

Continue to observe your emotions. Today I will ask you to do something a little bizarre. Take your favorite "guilt food" and eat it without emotion. Take the amount you would eat in an emotional moment. If it is a whole bag of Hershey® kisses (about 20 pieces) or a whole pint of ice cream, eat it. Be honest. Just doing this is already quite an experience because you will face a possible mountain of food on the table.

Buy it and sit down at a table on your own. Observe and analyze the ingredients if it is in a package. Eat slowly. (How long does it take to eat this if you do it mindfully?)

How does it taste? How much do you enjoy it? Maybe not at all when you are not emotional! Maybe you can't eat it all!

How do you feel after eating this? Do you notice anything regarding your body and mind? Do you observe stomach pain, lethargy, headache, brain fog, etc.?

Write down what you learned/observed:

Rationale and benefits of this experiment:
Eating a "guilty choice" without emotions may make you realize you don't like it as much or how much/how quickly you eat when in a mindless state. This will help you stop in your tracks next time.

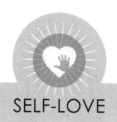

SELF-LOVE

Experiment #25 – Who Are You?

Write a mantra about yourself you can repeat silently or write on your computer or smart phone screen. You could leverage your artistic creativity and create a nice inspiring image to use as your screen wallpaper. Examples of personal mantras:

"I am a blooming flower."
"I am a beautiful person."
"I am in charge of me."

Write your self-love mantra:

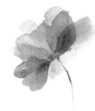

Rationale and benefits of this experiment:
When faced with a challenge, a setback, a lack of motivation, or a stressful event, take a few minutes to breathe in and out and repeat this mantra as long as you need. You are giving your mind and body a beautiful message of self-love and hope that will counteract whatever negative situation you are facing. It is a form of self-brainwashing, and it works! Because you will BELIEVE it!

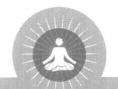

MINDFULNESS AND ZEN LIFE

Experiment #26 – Chewing Pounds Away

Be on your own for your next meal. Believe me this is important, because I will ask you to **chew at least 12 times** on each morsel you put in your mouth. You will want to do this, at least for the first time, in isolation!

Select a healthy and balanced meal with vegetables, a protein source, and a reasonable source of starchy carbohydrates such as potatoes or rice. You don't have to cook it yourself, but it is better if you do. You must be seated at a table. Block out a minimum of 30 minutes without interruptions.

Put your silverware back on the table after each bite. Measure your hunger and satiety levels regularly as you eat.

What do you notice when you chew each morsel 12 times?

_____

_____

_____

Rationale and benefits of this experiment:
You will realize a few things. For example, when we chew more, we eat less and feel satiated quicker. The idea is to help you learn to appreciate food. Chewing more slows you down, helps your digestion, and teaches you to be in the moment.

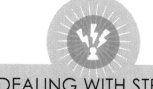

DEALING WITH STRESS

Experiment #27 – Kill the Energy Vampires

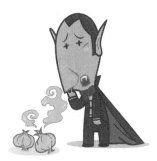

What happens when you are surrounded by negative energy created by people or situations? It stresses you out and takes away your own energy. Stress created by others impacts our bodies and minds. Some people are very good at creating drama by projecting their own stress on others. You need to learn to fight this, especially if stress triggers cravings.

There are three possible strategies:

1. Avoid the person/situation. Sometimes you have to say goodbye to energy vampires.
2. Minimize the encounters if you can't totally eliminate them.
3. Create a strategy to shield yourself from the vampire(s).
   a. Avoid discussion or confrontation.
   b. Ignore "the stressor" – continue to do what you were doing.
   c. Create a symbolic shield or bubble of protection around you. Imagine the negative energy bumping on this shield and not GETTING to you. You are in control. You are sending the negative vibes back.

Rationale and benefits of this experiment:
You will be surprised at the effectiveness of the "energy protective shield" methodology. You will get a kick out of it. After a few encounters, the energy vampire should start to change his or her behavior.

LIFE HACKS TO SIMPLIFY YOUR LIFE

Experiment #28 – Is Your Fitness Plan in Your Agenda?

Best way to not exercise or just move, is to let it happen as an afterthought. If you let your agenda be filled with activities, some not supporting your health quest, the chances are exercise will always get the boot first. This is especially true if you are not that excited, committed, or disciplined about it.

This week you are going to fill your calendar in 10-minute increments – as far as you can go – with specific time allocations for:

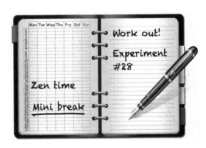

- Exercise or activity.
- Time to relax and be mindful.
- Time to do the CogniDiet® experiments.
- Mini mental breaks.

If you are not ready to do this, return to square one and ask yourself how committed you are to transformation. I don't want to be too tough, but you must start from somewhere. Start small, and then go bolder, but stick to the plan!

Rationale and benefits of this experiment:
Commitment in time is important to support a goal. We mark business meetings, doctor's appointments, and parties on our calendar, why not include everything that has to do with fitness?

Four Weeks Have Passed!
You Have Passed the Beginner Level

CONGRATULATIONS!

- You have been with me for four weeks.

- Old habits are starting to disappear.

- New healthier and more mindful habits are starting to appear.

- You must have learned a lot about yourself!

- Your body and mind have changed.

Enter the next four weeks with confidence or start over again if you feel you need a little more work.

- Do not forget to enter your key data and four-week statistics on page 7.

- Take a few pictures of yourself!

- Treat yourself with something nice! You deserve it.

Keep going!

The Advanced Level

Week 5

As we enter this week and graduated from the Beginner Level, the experiments are becoming more...let's say...challenging.

Continue to practice what you have learned. Enjoy your victories. You could have already lost four to 10 or more pounds if you:

1. Cut your calories by 20%.
2. Increased your activity level by even only 10%.
3. Cut the sugary snacks and drinks (includes alcohol).
4. Added vegetables in your life.
5. Took the time to love yourself more.
6. Realized the impact of stress and emotions on your behaviors.

Become even better and more committed now that you have built your healthy foundation.

Enter your data on page 7 and take your pictures.

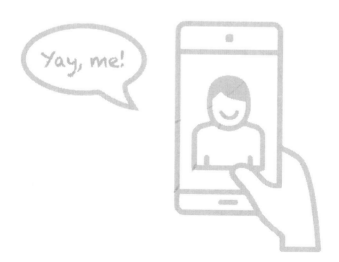

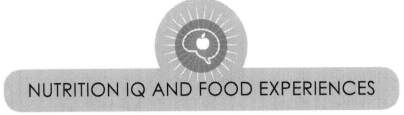

NUTRITION IQ AND FOOD EXPERIENCES

Experiment #29 – Shrink the Plate

We are asking you to downsize your plate or portions.

You can start by eating on dessert plates (in general they are the size of older regular plates). In the past, china plates were no more than 11″ in diameter. How big are yours? If you cannot find a smaller plate, take one of your regular plates, and mark 20% off the surface. Next time you use the plate, leave that 20% unfilled. However, once served, move the food all over the plate so it looks totally filled.

With the remaining surface, make sure half is always filled with non-starchy vegetables.

If you are not eating on a plate, such as when you have a slice of pizza at a pizza parlor, or are eating a sandwich, you can still play the 20% cut game.

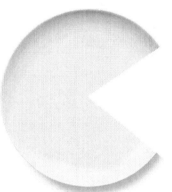

Rationale and benefits of this experiment:
Our eyes don't notice the difference between a large and a small plate. We eat what is on a plate. We finish it rather than listening to our hunger level. When we start to eat on a smaller plate or cut portions we will realize our hunger is satisfied.

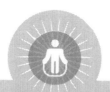

ACTIVITY LEVEL AND ENERGY

Experiment #30 – Do You Sweat Enough?

If you have not yet increased your activity level, you need to go back to the Beginner Level. Remember you are in Advanced Level now. You need activity for your health, not just for your weight loss. You need to use your arms and legs, you need to evacuate the stress. You need to eliminate hours spent in front of a screen.

We are a sedentary society. We have become immobile. This week your job is to lose at least one pound. Possibly more. I want you to sweat.

Are you really sweating when you exercise?

Last week we cut the plate or portion size. On Week 4 we asked you to increase your activity level by a minimum of 10%.

This week I want you to try a new activity just for fun. One that will make you sweat, get red and/or suffer more than usual.

- A new super-powered Zumba class.
- A free intro to the barre method.
- Start training for a 5K, 10K, half, or full marathon.

Rationale and benefits of this experiment:
If you are not sweating, you are not really burning calories optimally. Please be aware of your physical condition. I don't want you to have a heart attack!

EMOTIONS

Experiment #31 – Did I Really Eat This?

Remember **Experiment #24** last week about eating your guilty treat(s) mindfully? Next time you have an emotional meltdown, and you reach out to this same guilty treat, try to remember what triggered this, how you ate it, how you got access to it, and how you felt during and after eating it. Did it resolve the emotion by the way?

Now compare...

EVENT	MINDFUL EATING EXPERIMENT	EMOTIONAL EATING SITUATION	DO YOU SEE A FEW DIFFERENCES HERE?
EXAMPLE: I ate 12 sticks of Twizzler® after I felt sad.	What you learned last week:	What are you observing/feeling?	

Rationale and benefits of this experiment:

By comparing eating the same treat with or without emotions you can realize how much you really like the treat, or not, and how differently and mindlessly you shove food through your throat when in the grasp of an emotion.

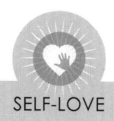

SELF-LOVE

Experiment #32 – I Love You Because...

This is a little unnerving. It requires courage. Ask three family members and three good friends to tell you, via a letter or email, what they love most about you (at every level: morally, spiritually, personality-wise, and physically).

Last week my husband told me I was so good at summarizing complicated stories or situations. This came as a surprise to me. I did not know that. It made me feel good.

Make sure when collected that you keep this feedback preciously, reflect upon it and enjoy it!

Dear friend,
What I love about you...

Rationale and benefits of this experiment:
It is always good to hear and read what people think and believe about us. Very often our loved ones, out of education, personality, or habit will not laud us with compliments. We tend to focus more on shortcomings, and that focus erodes our self-confidence.

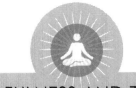

MINDFULNESS AND ZEN LIFE

Experiment #33 – Is It Good Enough for Me?

Next time you feel you may be tempted remember you can leave the situation (out of sight, out of mind), use visualization (**Experiment #12**), recite your mantra (**Experiment #25**), or use breathing techniques (**Experiment #20**).

If you feel nothing is working, I believe it is because you are not practicing these techniques enough.

Here is yet another way of dealing with a temptation. Ask yourself three questions:

1. **Is this so unique** that not eating it will be one of my life's regrets? Yes, of course if you were at a three-star Michelin restaurant!
2. **Is this so delicious** that I should really have at least a bite or two?
3. **Am I so hungry** (count to 10 and gauge this) that if I do not eat, I will faint? And if I am so hungry, is this the kind of food I should eat anyhow?

If none of these questions gets a YES, why eat this? It must be plain and forgettable food. And you are not even hungry!

Rationale and benefits of this experiment:
Questioning the food you face gets your logical brain to really observe the food almost scientifically. To summarize, you learn to say: "Is it good enough for me?" This will stop you in your tracks and take the impulsiveness away.

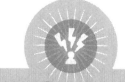

DEALING WITH STRESS

Experiment #34 – The Beautification Project

Have you surrounded yourself with soothing elements such as nice pictures, an aromatherapy diffuser, a salt lamp, meditation beads, flowers, or a beautiful object of art?

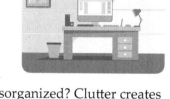

What does your office, cubicle, or desk look like? Is it messy, full of papers, disorganized? Clutter creates stress. Clutter eats up energy. Stress triggers cravings. You need and deserve an inspiring and calming environment.

Action: Take the place where you spend most time during the day. Assess the look, feel, beauty factor, tidiness, and inspirational factor. Then make a few changes that support your new journey. It does not have to be expensive!

Rationale and benefits of this experiment:
Your environment impacts your senses of sight, sound, and smell, therefore your mood. A dirty desk in a noisy office, with nothing personal and inspiring is not going to make you happy. On the other hand, looking at something beautiful creates positivity. If you, like many people, only have only a small cubicle, you can still include something personal. If you never know where you will sit, carry something nice with you.

LIFE HACKS TO SIMPLIFY YOUR LIFE

Experiment #35 – Pantry Tsunami

Have you cleaned out your pantries, office drawers, and car of unneeded food? Do you still have secret stashes in your house? If you eliminate the temptations, you will stop thinking about them.

Do you have loving saboteurs at home (see Chapter 7 in *Weight Loss Starts in Your Brain*). If so, create special storage places just for them. Give your partner or children a special drawer for their cookies. I have a client who stored the ice cream and sweets for her children in the basement. It was out of sight and far away! She noticed a decline in snacking in the household.

Remember the more there is in your pantry, freezer, and fridge, the more food will be consumed in your home. Buying in bulk is more economical, but do you need such large quantities at home? Unless you have five growing kids to feed, I doubt it.

Action: This week clean and decide what is essential, must stay and is aligned with your journey to health. Whatever is too sugary, too artificial, too fattening, or outdated must go.

Rationale and benefits of this experiment:
You need to surround yourself, at every level, with things to support the lifestyle you desire to achieve. Everything that is not, will work against you.

Week 6

You are getting close. You are almost halfway into your self-discovery journey.

Have you cleaned your pantry, beautified your work environment and gotten the feedback about yourself from your friends?

Remember the importance of your environment and self-perception in supporting or sabotaging your efforts to change.

I hope a feeling of freedom from dieting is invading your mood. I wish you are discovering wonderful things about yourself, because there are many things about ourselves that are amazing.

Are you enjoying your new "skinnier" plate? Have you noticed how much less you eat and still not feel hungry?

To tell you a little secret, **Experiment #33** is one I use all the time when personally faced with temptations, it really works!

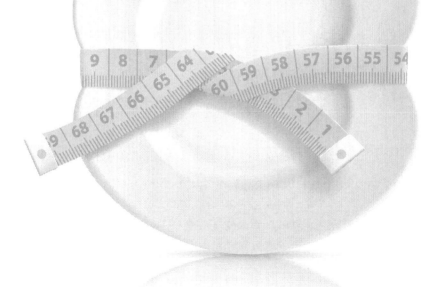

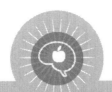

NUTRITION IQ AND FOOD EXPERIENCES

Experiment #36 – The Breakfast Challenge

This experiment is to make you aware of what an overload of sugar, including what very high glycemic index carbohydrates can do to your glucose level, and therefore to future sugar cravings. Remember the more sugar you eat, the more you will want it. **This is not an experiment for people with diabetes or blood sugar issues.**

One morning, have a breakfast quite high in sugar and white carbohydrates: white toast, muffins, or commercial cereals with fat free milk, jam, fruit juice.

Next day, have a more balanced meal that combines carbohydrates with fat and protein, such as ham, tofu, eggs, and nut butters, etc.

Observe how you feel until lunchtime:
- Do you crave for sugar or carbohydrates?
- Do you feel hungry?
- Are you feeling energetic and focused?

Cogni-Tip: Make sure you read Chapter 2 on sugar in *Weight Loss Starts in Your Brain.* It explains the rules about combining fat, protein and carbohydrates to avoid sugar cravings. It is called "linking."

Rationale and benefits of this experiment:
By doing this experiment you become more aware of what sugar does to you, including your ability to focus and feel energized.

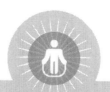

ACTIVITY LEVEL AND ENERGY

Experiment #37 – Plan an Adventure Trip

I will encourage you this week to plan, book, or just embark ASAP on a special active trip with loved one(s).

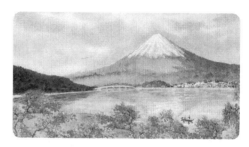

Are you going on a two-hour kayaking adventure, a three-day mountain climb, a day beach trip, or a one-week volcano discovery? The activity does not matter.

Combine the activity with relaxation and nature. This is different from going to the gym or meeting with a trainer.

This is planning a trip with an activity focus, rather than just the plain old resort or family home trip. This does not mean you are not active while on holiday! But this is a trip with an activity goal which is very different.

Put something on your calendar this weekend. No excuses. Find strategies to make it happen. If on a tight budget, plan something local. There is always a park or a beach you can access for free.

Rationale and benefits of this experiment:
This is the transformational experience. This is how you change your lifestyle. Your life becomes more focused on being on the move and enjoying it. Moving is the antidote to aging.

EMOTIONS

Experiment #38 – My Wants

In *Weight Loss Starts in Your Brain*, we explore what is behind your emotions. Once you start to observe and de-construct your major emotions you must be able to realize emotions are better dealt with if you describe their root cause and how they can be fixed. Because then you can act!

Example: "I feel very lonely because I have no friends. Therefore, out of sadness, I drown myself in Twinkies®."

Let's ask the person who wrote this to write his or her **WANTS**. An emotion is a physical feeling. The expression of a WANT is a path to action:

- I want to be loved and appreciated.
- I want to have fun with friends.
- I want to have a social life.

Action: How can you change that? What are the root causes of your isolation? Maybe it is time to get out of your shell, call friends, invite people over, join a club, or discover new activities.

Select your top emotions and de-construct them in the same way. Then make an action plan.

EMOTION	MY WANTS
#1	
#2	
#3	
#4	
#5	
#6	

 Rationale and benefits of this experiment:
It is important to face your emotions even when they are painful. If you use food to numb your emotions, you will never resolve them and will continue to eat them. This is a tough experiment that may require some psychological professional support.

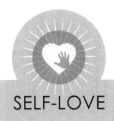

SELF-LOVE

Experiment #39 – My Achievements

Write a list of your life's many accomplishments. I am not talking about talents or skills. I am talking about a list of things you are proud of and should not hesitate to boast about.

- I have an engineering degree.
- I am debt-free.
- I was a cross country state champion in Nevada in my teens.
- I won an award for _____ at the office.
- I started a company at 20.
- I am independent financially.
- I can run one mile in 10 minutes and I am 50 years old.

You can also reflect on your past weight loss successes. It may be surprising I added this on the list, but you did a lot of things to lose the weight. Remember them.

Write your list: _____

_____

_____

Rationale and benefits of this experiment:
We tend to always feel we could have or should have done more. We are focused on the future and don't spend enough time reflecting on the past. By making that list you will realize how great you are. This confidence will boost your future endeavors.

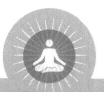

MINDFULNESS AND ZEN LIFE

Experiment #40 – My Body Is a Temple

This week splurge in a Zen or spiritual-like activity that forces you to at least spend a half day away from people, tasks, and phones. I am not talking about a forest bath or a kayaking adventure. This is more of an alternative healing and holistic journey.

A few mindful experiences to enhance your relaxation level:

- A guided meditation session with a teacher.
- A spa experience such as a salt water floatation therapy or a few hours in a Himalayan salt cave.
- Time with a Reiki expert or energy healer.
- Drum circles.

This is about recharging your batteries with a mindful experience. If you have zero budget, rest on a nice sofa, get a free guided meditation on YouTube® (there are plenty), and just do it with focus. No interruptions!

Rationale and benefits of this experiment:
This type of experiment will bring you to a state of happiness and contentment that will boost happy neurotransmitters and promote wellbeing. When you are happy and relaxed, cravings may not occur!

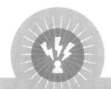

DEALING WITH STRESS

Experiment #41 – My Secret Stress Eraser

We don't always have the luxury of disappearing and isolating ourselves when stress hits. Here are a few objects you can wear or carry that may help calm you down. They can be secret or on plain view on your desk. I have a Himalayan salt bowl with balls of salt in it that when heated feel very soothing and warm in my hands. Here are a few suggestions:

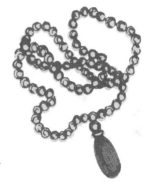

- A squishy ball or object.
- Praying or mantra beads worn as a bracelet or necklace.
- A secret object hidden in your pocket, like a stone or a personal meaningful talisman.

The idea is you have to be able to touch and play with the object.

Rationale and benefits of this experiment:
The secret (or discreet) object you carry helps deflect the stress by way of your hand(s) expelling it through the action of squeezing or rubbing. Or the counting the beads will help calm down your brain through the repetition of a gesture. Don't forget to breathe!

LIFE HACKS TO SIMPLIFY YOUR LIFE

Experiment #42 – Am I High Maintenance?

How much time do you spend grooming yourself? Are you a
high maintenance kind of person? This can be true for men, too.
Include in your list manicures, pedicures, blow outs, hair styling,
makeup, waxing, lashes tinting or extensions, fillers injections,
facials, and shopping for new clothes.

Rate yourself on a scale from 1 (low maintenance) to 10
(extremely high maintenance).

LOW MAINTENANCE ○ ○ ○ ○ ○ ○ ○ ○ ○ ○ EXTREMELY HIGH MAINTENANCE
1 2 3 4 5 6 7 8 9 10

Write a list of what can be eliminated. This is different from
Experiment #14 because here you are simplifying your
"grooming" regimen.

I am spending $_____ a month on personal grooming.

I am spending _____ hours a month on personal grooming.

I can let go of _____

I can downsize _____

Rationale and benefits of this experiment:
*This helps you continue to eliminate things in the way
of your goals. I call them the time vampires. Maybe one
less blow dry a week will free you up to go to the gym
one more hour or buy a new bike.*

Week 7

You are halfway done. You did six weeks already.

Are there any experiments you wish to redo? Maybe it is time to take a break and go backward.

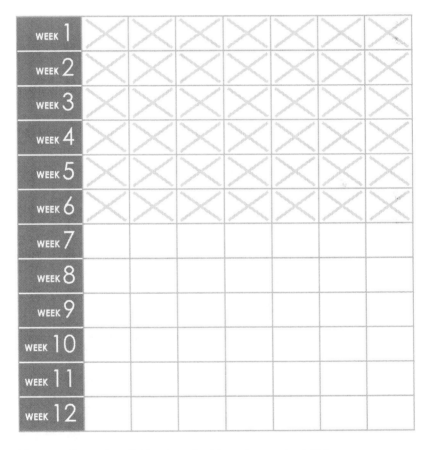

You continue to eliminate what is not needed. This was a very self-oriented week. You are treating yourself with spiritual gifts. You are taking care of yourself by prioritizing activities that serve your quest for a healthier life.

Have you booked this adventure trip yet?

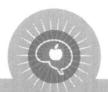

NUTRITION IQ AND FOOD EXPERIENCES

Experiment #43 – Vegetables First

Please start to eat your lunch or dinner with a salad and non-starchy vegetables. Then, and only when these have been eaten, can you eat your protein and starchy carbohydrates such as fries, bread, rice, potatoes, or pasta.

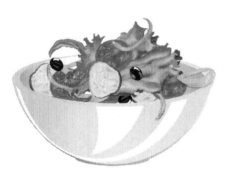

In addition to a starter salad, vegetables should still cover 50% of your plate surface.

Note your appetite and hunger level after you have eaten all these vegetables.

Rationale and benefits of this experiment:

Vegetables require more chewing, unless in a puree form, than starchy carbohydrates. They also contain more water, especially if raw. They will occupy more volume in your stomach. There will be less room left for the rest of the food. Therefore, you will eat less and feel full quicker.

In the future start with vegetables, a lot of them. They will also stabilize your glucose level and provide fiber. They will help control, and even potentially avoid future cravings.

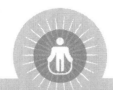

ACTIVITY LEVEL AND ENERGY

Experiment #44 – Discover a New Activity

Sometimes the brain needs a shock, something new to trigger a new behavior. Always exercising with the same routine renders your muscle mass and metabolism lazier because they become accustomed to the same old moves.

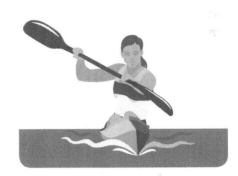

I congratulate you for your increased level of activity. Bravo. Maybe it is now time to embark on something you have been thinking about for a while but have not tried. It may be a Zumba dancing class, or a spin class. It could be you want to try something to help with flexibility, stress relief, or meditation.

It must be something you never did before. What can it be? Ask friends, inquire at your gym if you have a membership, or explore online programs.

I will try _____

_____

Rationale and benefits of this experiment:
We all need novelty and change occasionally. Exercise routines can become boring. Boredom becomes an excuse for not exercising anymore.

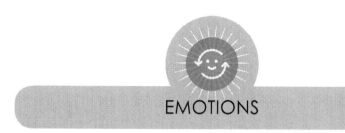

EMOTIONS

Experiment #45 – Time to Have a Tough Conversation

Remember energy vampires (**Experiment #27**) and all that you
have accomplished so far to get to the bottom of your emotions.

This week, be brave. There must be a few emotions that impact
the way you are being perceived or treated by certain persons.

One way to deal with an emotion is to get at the root of it and
deal with it. Some emotions are rooted in past experiences,
abuse, or trauma and must be dealt with the help of professional
healthcare practitioners.

I am talking about something that could be easily fixed via
a conversation. Here is a personal example. At one point my
mother was always criticizing the way I dressed. It made me feel
"not good enough," not the perfect daughter, etc. Until the point
when I said to myself: "why should I care about what she thinks.
Sometimes I don't like the way she dresses, too."

So, I talked to her. She still makes comments, but nothing
compared to the amount she used to make. I look at her with my
death stare when she starts. I expressed my WANTS (remember
Experiment #38).

Write down situations you want to address and prepare your
conversations. Writing down what you want to express is
very important. Be specific, fact-based, and speak from your
perspective. Be clear about the reasons why you want a change.

Use words like "I need," "this is what I want," "this is the way it
must work," etc.

Here are my wants:

Rationale and benefits of this experiment:

You will be surprised at how liberating and easy it is to say what YOU WANT. This will be one less emotion that triggered a craving because you chose not to express yourself.

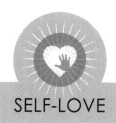

SELF-LOVE

Experiment #46 – Mirror, Mirror!

Every morning when you are ready, but before you leave home, look at yourself in the mirror and give yourself a compliment. We all have the habit, especially women, to always focus on what we do not have, what is wrong with us, or what we could do better. This usually has to do with our physical appearances.

We could be thinner, larger breasted, flatter chested, or have longer legs, etc. In **Experiments #4** and **#11**, we asked you to describe your best intellectual, moral, personality, and physical assets.

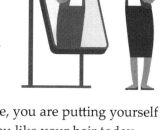

We want you to focus on the positives. You are gorgeous as you are.

By giving yourself a nice smile and a compliment before you leave the house, you are putting yourself into a positive state of mind. Maybe you like your hair today, did a great job with the eye makeup, or love your new dress.

Rationale and benefits of this experiment:
First, smiling, including to yourself, is known to give a happy little boost to your brain. Secondly, leaving the house in a positive frame of mind will set the tone and confidence you feel for the whole day as it unfolds.

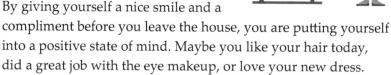

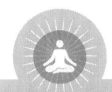

MINDFULNESS AND ZEN LIFE

Experiment #47 – Are You in the Moment?

Take any moment in the day or the week but try to choose a time where you are not working.

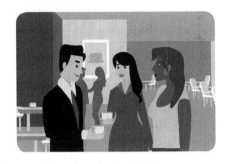

Select a time when you are with your children, family, or friends. Before the event, decide you will be 100% there. You will not be thinking about how you look, how people may feel about you, or what you need to do tomorrow.

Just be present and in the moment 100%. Notice the details: The voices. The conversations. The décor. Observe people's faces and gestures in a non-judgmental manner. Appreciate whatever is happening: a dinner, a game, an event, etc. Feel how happy you are to be there.

When you come home, reflect on the moment. Were you there really 100%, at least for most of the time? Being in the moment and enjoying the company, is usually a great diverter from food temptation.

Rationale and benefits of this experiment:
Being in the moment and appreciating what is going on is the best way to combat the unrelenting low-level stress we usually experience. By going with the flow and being present, you enjoy life to the fullest.

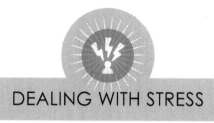

DEALING WITH STRESS

Experiment #48 – Short Term Stress Elimination

We learned about our stress levels, and whether or not a situation is unbearable. We learned about the need to relax and find ways to make our brain happy with visualization (**Experiment #12**) or breathing mindfully (**Experiment #20**).

Today we are talking about creating an elimination list. There are long-term issues, such as an awful commute or a difficult marriage, that require long term planning and do need to be addressed. There are also short-term issues that can be easily fixed to lower your stress factor.

Are you on too many committees or charity boards? Are you trying to squeeze too much in your agenda? Write the list of stress-creating ACTIVITIES you can eliminate NOW. You already eliminated at least one in Week 1. Eliminate at least three to five more now.

I eliminate: _____

_____

_____

Rationale and benefits of this experiment:
There is no point in saying you are stressed out if you put yourself in these situations. You can only handle what is bearable to you. Some people can handle more than others. There is no shame in limiting some activities. You will become more productive.

LIFE HACKS TO SIMPLIFY YOUR LIFE

Experiment #49 – Simplify or Just Start Cooking

The CogniDiet® supports cooking and eating fresh and balanced foods, but not everybody has the time, nor desire to cook, especially every day.

Let me emphasize that eating at restaurants and buying take-out, even if convenient, is both more expensive and always higher in calories, fats, sugars, and salt content than home-cooking.

Considering recent lifestyle trends, grocery shops and chains have adapted and offer more possibilities than ever to buy semi-peeled, spiralized, chopped, frozen, or cooked foods. All you have to do is reheat the food or do some minor cooking.

If you are one of the people who after six weeks is still struggling to nourish herself or himself properly and continues to rely on processed, packaged, and fast foods, this experiment is for you. Buy a prepared bundle of fresh foods and cook today or this weekend. There are also reasonably priced companies delivering uncooked meals.

Note how long it took. Is this such a challenge?

Rationale and benefits of this experiment:
You need to be in control of what you eat, and cooking at home is one of the best ways to do so. Freezing portions or keeping leftovers is one way to stretch the cooking for a few days. Just give it a try.

Week 8

This was a demanding week! You had a lot to do. You have been pushed hard.

Having a tough conversation with a loved one(s) is not easy, but you have the right to put yourself FIRST.

Yes, we are very pro-vegetables at The CogniDiet® because we believe they deliver many health benefits and help you control cravings.

The "Eat Your Vegetables First" or **Experiment #43** is essential, as well as the one you did on Week 6 with the breakfast challenge (**Experiment #36**). Don't you feel better and more in control?

How are you feeling today?

Write it down: _____

_____

_____

_____

_____

_____

_____

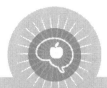

NUTRITION IQ AND FOOD EXPERIENCES

Experiment #50 – No Snacks Needed

You already cut calories by cutting snacks in Week 1, remember, you are supposed to stick to that. Snacks can easily add 500 to 1,000 calories a day before we know it.

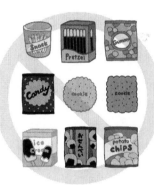

You do not need snacks if you eat regularly and well. Snacks have been invented by the food industry to make you eat more. Why do you think they are transportable and in single-use packages?

This week I am asking you to stop all snacking activities. Even the few nuts at 10 am, and the apple at 4 pm. Do you really need them? Are you hungry? Are you going to faint if you don't eat them?

If not, you do not need these snacks. They have become a habit. Even food diaries now have entries for am and pm snacks. Just having this entry in a diary gives you permission to have snacks.

As you embark on this new level of food self-control, notice how much weight you lose this week. Do you notice an acceleration? If you are not a "snacker" at all, watch your portions. Maybe they are still too large.

Rationale and benefits of this experiment:
You are in weight loss acceleration mode now. Snacking is one of the major reasons people do not lose weight.

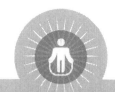

ACTIVITY LEVEL AND ENERGY

Experiment #52 – Snap Out of It!

There is not always time to stop, ponder, and do some soul searching when an emotion hits and you immediately crave chocolate.

By this eighth week you should be more familiar with your emotions and what triggers them. I hope you also know a cookie will not solve it. On the contrary, a cookie will trigger another emotion called guilt and a sense of failure, which will then trigger a new craving followed by a new sense of failure and zero self-worth. This is the vicious circle of emotional eating.

While you work on solutions, sometimes it is easier to just "snap out of it."

Pause, and physically snap your fingers, tap on your wrist (some people wear an elastic band), or give yourself an imaginary or real face slap. And say to yourself:

"Snap out of it darling, it will pass." Then move on. Tell yourself you will deal with the emotion later!

Rationale and benefits of this experiment:
This experiment allows you to perform a noticeable physical and/or mental action that will give you a little shock. The shock will be enough to distract you from the cookie and realize it is not a solution to your emotion.

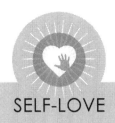

SELF-LOVE

Experiment #53 – Don't Be a Wallflower

This is about confidence boosting. This is about being daring, unabashedly, and unapologetically. I am asking you to do something you have never done before because you are afraid of people's reaction, of what they may think of you.

Of course we care about other people's opinions and judgment. Often, we inhibit ourselves by creating hypothetical limits or boundaries on our actions or behaviors, based on supposed opinions:

- She will think I am a fool.
- He will think I am too sexy in that dress.
- They will make fun of my new hat.
- I am "too fat" to wear a swimsuit at the beach, people will think I am a whale.

Well my friends, let me tell you: People don't care.

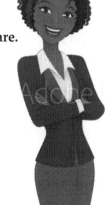

This week, or soon, you will wear or do something new. You lost 10 pounds and bought a new dress that is slightly sexier? WEAR IT. And then observe the environment. I guarantee you most people will not notice—or will pay you a compliment.

Rationale and benefits of this experiment:
This experiment is meant to boost self-confidence and independence of spirit! Just flaunt the new you.

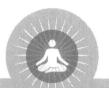

MINDFULNESS AND ZEN LIFE

Experiment #54 – Have a Mindful Dinner

In this experiment we are asking you to plan and take the time to set up a nice lunch or dinner, on your own, or with company. Here are the rules:

- You must be part of the planning, including the menu, which must be healthy. Dessert and wine are acceptable.
- The dinner must be seated, the table must be well decorated and attractive. Make it beautiful with nice linens, candles, your best silverware, china, and flowers, etc.
- It is better if you are not involved with the cooking and serving. It could be in a restaurant, but that might be too noisy, or they could push you out too soon.
- Before dinner starts, please say something, it can be silent, to express your gratitude for the food that will nourish you today.
- Decide you will enjoy every morsel, slowly, and deliberately. Remember to chew more than three times before you swallow, ideally 12 times. After each morsel, put down your silverware.
- Appreciate the colors, textures, smells, and flavors with each bite.
- Ignore the pace and how others are eating, just focus on your own experience. You can also enjoy the conversation but keep it light and pleasant.

After the meal, write down your experience.

Rationale and benefits of this experiment:
This experience is meant to develop your appreciation of slow eating.

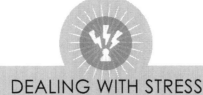

DEALING WITH STRESS

Experiment #55 – Find Your #1 Way to De-stress

Everybody has different ways to unwind. Some methods work better for some than others. You may be completely calm after walking in nature, while somebody else may need an hour of kick-boxing.

Is there something you have not yet explored? I know what calms me down is anything in nature or linked to water.

If and when you have discovered it, practice it at least three times a week or everyday if it only requires a few minutes (like meditation). It is imperative to stick to what works best for you. It could be a combination of things, such as running, and meditation like me. And by the way, these are both free activities.

My #1 Way to De-stress is: _____

_____

I will devote _____ hours/days to its practice every week.

Rationale and benefits of this experiment:
By sticking to what you prefer, and what delivers the best results, you increase your chances of providing what is best to your overdriven brain. Make sure you eliminate what is not needed, such as the yoga class you attend to appease your friend but that you don't like so much – in fact it stresses you out.

LIFE HACKS TO SIMPLIFY YOUR LIFE

Experiment #56 – Describe Your Day

When you look at your day, even the past few days, how do
you slice the way you spent it? Let's play that game. Enter the
activities in 30-minute increments. However, if you take a 10
or 15-minute mental break, note that, too. If you eat in only 10
minutes, please note it.

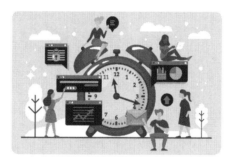

Start as early and stop as late as you want to reflect on your
typical schedule. A little comment however. I hope you are
sleeping at least seven to eight hours a night. It is important for
your health, brain power, mental balance and weight loss.

Rationale and benefits of this experiment:
*This experiment's goal is to make you aware of how
you spend your days. Is there wasted or duplicated
time? Is it organized in a way that supports your health
goals? Do you allocate enough time to mini mental
breaks? What could be changed? It is recommended to
do the experiment for several days in a row to show a
behavioral trend. Then try to remediate.*

MY DAY

5 AM	5:15 AM	5:30 AM	5:45 AM	6 AM

6 AM	6:15 AM	6:30 AM	6:45 AM	7 AM

7 AM	7:15 AM	7:30 AM	7:45 AM	8 AM

8 AM	8:15 AM	8:30 AM	8:45 AM	9 AM

9 AM	9:15 AM	9:30 AM	9:45 AM	10 AM

10 AM	10:15 AM	10:30 AM	10:45 AM	11 AM

11 AM	11:15 AM	11:30 AM	11:45 AM	12 PM

12 PM	12:15 PM	12:30 PM	12:45 PM	1 PM

1 PM	1:15 PM	1:30 PM	1:45 PM	2 PM

2 PM	2:15 PM	2:30 PM	2:45 PM	3 PM

3 PM	3:15 PM	3:30 PM	3:45 PM	4 PM

4 PM	4:15 PM	4:30 PM	4:45 PM	5 PM

MY NIGHT

5 PM	5:15 PM	5:30 PM	5:45 PM	6 PM

6 PM	6:15 PM	6:30 PM	6:45 PM	7 PM

7 PM	7:15 PM	7:30 PM	7:45 PM	8 PM

8 PM	8:15 PM	8:30 PM	8:45 PM	9 PM

9 PM	9:15 PM	9:30 PM	9:45 AM	10 AM

10 PM	10:15 PM	10:30 PM	10:45 PM	11 PM

11 PM	11:15 PM	11:30 PM	11:45 PM	12 AM

12 AM	12:15 AM	12:30 AM	12:45 AM	1 AM

1 AM	1:15 AM	1:30 AM	1:45 AM	2 AM

2 AM	2:15 AM	2:30 AM	2:45 AM	3 AM

3 AM	3:15 AM	3:30 AM	3:45 AM	4 AM

4 AM	4:15 AM	4:30 AM	4:45 AM	5 AM

Eight Weeks Have Passed!
You Have Passed the Advanced Level

CONGRATULATIONS!

- You have undertaken 56 experiments!

- You must have learned a lot about yourself!

- Have you realized the environment is starting to align around your mission and vision for yourself?

- How are people around you reacting?

- What is your confidence level?

- You must be an inspiration to others, what did they tell you about your transformation?

I lost _____ pounds in the past eight weeks.

Enter the last four weeks with confidence or start over again if you feel you need to work a little bit more. Do not hesitate to repeat experiments.

- Enter your key data and eight-week statistics on page 7.

- Take a few pictures of yourself!

- Treat yourself with something even nicer! You deserve it.

Almost there

THE FINAL FOUR WEEKS

The Master Level

Week 9

The Last Stretch to Master Level!

Don't forget to take your picture and enter your data!

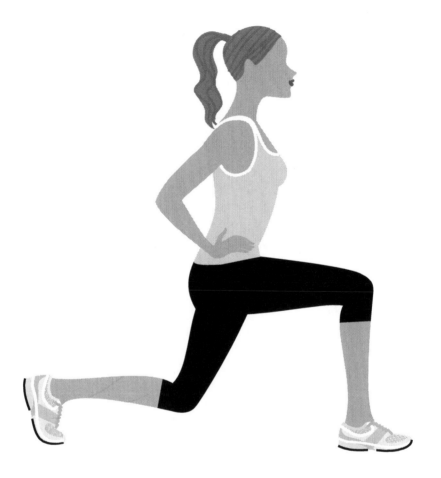

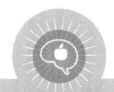

NUTRITION IQ AND FOOD EXPERIENCES

Experiment #57 – Count Your Bites

This week, become aware of how many bites you put in your mouth. This is a good and practical way to calculate how much you eat and avoid the need for a calorie counter or app. Though, you could use one too (good ones are MyFitnessPal and Lose It!).

Use the following rules:

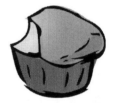

- Each bite is approximately 30 calories.
- If the bite is heavy in fat or sugar, count it as 50 calories (yes, it is possible).
- If it is vegetables, it is usually 10 calories.

If you want to simplify, use an average of 30 calories. If you do not feel doing this during meals, do it at least in-between, when snacking occurs here and there, often mindlessly.

My bites today were _____

This is equal to _____ calories.

Go back to *Weight Loss Starts in Your Brain*, Chapter 4," My Body is a Temple with Limited Square Feet," and calculate what you should eat in general. Are you exceeding your budget?

Rationale and benefits of this experiment:
This experiment's goal is to make you aware of how many times you put food in your mouth, sometimes unconsciously. Also, it means one bite plus another bite plus another bite can end up representing an extra 500 calories!

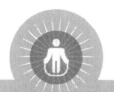

ACTIVITY LEVEL AND ENERGY

Experiment #58 – Record and Admire Your Progress

What did you enter into the grid capturing your body evolution on page 7? Do you notice more definition in your calves? Has your waist shrunk? What has changed in your face?

By now you should have lost eight to 16 pounds, possibly more. This is at least one or two dress or pants sizes down!

Write down the differences you observe in your body, not just the numbers, but also the appearance, the firmness factor, and the definition of the muscles, etc. Be descriptive and use your imagination.

I have noticed _____

_____

_____

_____

Rationale and benefits of this experiment:
This experiment is meant to make you appreciate and internalize the progress you have made and the results you have achieved. Writing them down makes them tangible. Note that any progress is progress. Some of us are quicker than others. You are not comparing yourself to anybody.

EMOTIONS

Experiment #59 – Create a Distractions List

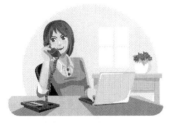

The way we progress is by staying focused on our mission. If and when you are still struggling with a temptation, the five-second "snap-out-of-it-method," or the breathing methods may not be appropriate.

Sometimes a simple but effective distraction will engage your brain in another direction and hopefully it will forget about the temptation.

- Engage in an activity that requires moving (go for a walk with a purpose).
- Engage your brain with something other than the thought of food which requires full attention: a telephone call, a conversation, or a mental activity such as sudoku, etc.
- Distract your brain with an unexpected sense-related experience such as drinking water, smelling diffused aromatic oils (citrusy plants, lavender and minty smells are perfect), eating something bitter, minty, or acidic.

Rationale and benefits of this experiment:
You will start to develop alternative strategies to cope with emotional cravings. Usually the brain will forget about the craving after a few minutes. The secret is to be 100% engaged in the other activity so it has to be meaningful and deliberate.

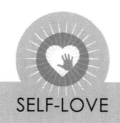

SELF-LOVE

Experiment #60 – Learn to Forgive Yourself and Move On

We are imperfect and perfectly beautiful as we are. Nobody is perfect all the time. We incur setbacks, we face obstacles, and we have to deal with saboteurs. We struggle. Even Gisele Bundchen, the famous Brazilian model struggles.

This week I want you to learn to forgive yourself and move on after a setback. Was it a giant cheesecake and margaritas at the party last weekend? Is it that you still succumb to ice cream when faced with it? Our brain is never going to forget the taste of sugar. This is a fact. But you can learn to tame the beast.

Next time you encounter a setback, instead of blaming yourself and self-sabotaging your future, write yourself a love note, and an action plan. As an example:

"I had ice cream last night, way too much. I enjoyed it but then realized I was bingeing. It was not so much the ice cream I enjoyed. I went into a mechanical eating pattern. **I am forgiving myself**. It happens. Tough life. Rome was not built in a day. Let's move on and avoid having ice cream at home. Today I will pay particular attention to my diet."

Rationale and benefits of this experiment:
Learning to write words such as "I forgive myself" is very important. You must eliminate the guilt factor. Own your indulgences and move on. Guilt is just a negative and unproductive emotion.

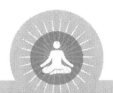

MINDFULNESS AND ZEN LIFE

Experiment #61 – Write Your Vision Movie Scenario

Remember when you learned to visualize a movie you had created to calm your brain and make it happy when you were stressed? You wrote the first script in **Experiment #12** in Week 2. It involved a moment in your life, or several, when you felt happiness at the highest level, in perfect harmony with the world and yourself. You made it as vivid as possible, using all of your senses. It did not have to be a long movie, just one scene was enough. I hope you have used it with great results.

Now you have evolved. I bet even your self-vision has changed. Maybe it is time to write a new inspiring scenario. Let's imagine YOU as a Zen-like, happy, grounded, and liberated from diets healthy individual.

Where are you? What are you wearing? What are you doing? Who are you with? Feel the happiness factor, the joy, the aura around you, your contagious laughter and energy. FEEL, FEEL, FEEL.

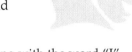

Now write your vision story, always starting with the word "I".

Rationale and benefits of this experiment:
Writing a movie about your vision, and making it real in your brain, at least once a day, will solidify your mission to change. Imagining what you want to be will help you become it.

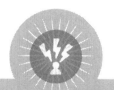

DEALING WITH STRESS

Experiment #62 – Leave Your Worries in a Box

Every night before going to bed, write what
stresses you out, things that you have not been
able or willing to fix yet, or something that
really hurt you that day.

Don't go to sleep with a stressed out or
angry mind. It will sabotage a good night's
sleep. You need sleep (read Chapter 11 page
281 in *Weight Loss Starts in Your Brain*) to give your brain a break.
You will continue to rehash the events and situations in your
head instead of going to sleep. It will even affect your dreams.

Instead, get a nice box, let's call it the "Worry Box" that you leave
outside your bedroom. Write down the situation, in details, on
a piece of paper, and leave it in the box, deciding to deal with it
the next day. Tonight, enter your bedroom and fall asleep in total
serenity.

Remember **Experiment #13** in Week 2 when we asked you to rate
the stress level of a situation. You could also give a severity rating
to the problems you are thinking about. I bet the next day the
rating will come down!

Rationale and benefits of this experiment:
*Writing about a problem or an issue is a way of taking
care of it. In fact, a good night of sleep can deliver a nice
solution in the morning. In the evening, you are tired,
and it is never a good time to think about problems.*

LIFE HACKS TO SIMPLIFY YOUR LIFE

Experiment #63 – Clean Your Wardrobe

By now you should feel a difference in your clothes. You may have lost one or two sizes. Keeping clothes you will never wear again keeps positive energy away from your goals.

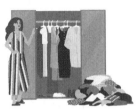

Divide your wardrobe in three sections:
1. What you never want to wear ever again (items that are too big).
2. What you are wearing now, that fits you almost perfectly.
3. What is yet too small, or that you wore when you were 19.

Section 1 must disappear. It releases negative energy. It silently tells you these clothes are there for you if and when you gain weight again. But you have no intention to go there again.

Section 2 must stay.

Section 3 can be kept for a while as you continue to lose weight. The smaller sized clothes make you feel inadequate and a failure. They tell you: "I will never fit in my prom dress again." These are negative thoughts. Get rid of them, too. Only keep what is reasonable in terms of size, style, and quality.

Cogni-Tip: A tailor can only fix a garment one size, maybe two sizes down. It is expensive, and you may never recover the perfect cut of the cloth.

Rationale and benefits of this experiment:
This is a life hack because it moves negative energy out of your environment.

Week 10

Only three weeks left. Have you cleaned out your wardrobe yet? I know it could take some time. As Marie Kondo, "clothes-purger" extraordinaire, advises "If you don't feel love as you hold the cloth or the object, don't keep it."

Remember, it is all about making room for your transformation to take place.

Take a pen and draw your weight loss curve to see where it is going. Highlight a trend.

WEIGHT:

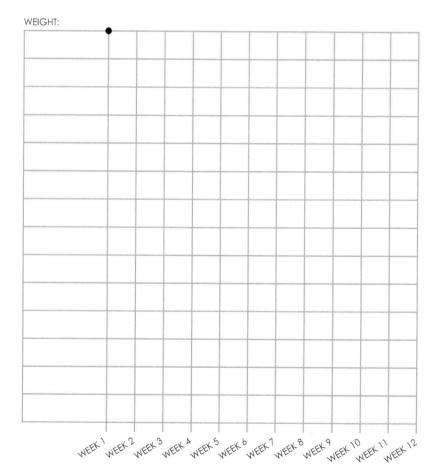

WEEK 1 WEEK 2 WEEK 3 WEEK 4 WEEK 5 WEEK 6 WEEK 7 WEEK 8 WEEK 9 WEEK 10 WEEK 11 WEEK 12

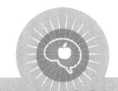

NUTRITION IQ AND FOOD EXPERIENCES

Experiment #64 – Use Your Eyes

By now you should be able to estimate what is on your plate. We recommend using apps such as "MyFitnessPal" or "Lose It!" to learn how to estimate and track your macros. But you also must become good at eyeing what is on your plate without these. Here are what you will use this week to estimate your plate.

Warning: These are approximations, but will be very helpful when trying to quickly assess what is in your plate:
- Vegetables: cooked - one cup equals +/- 30-40 calories, uncooked - one cup equals +/- 20 calories.
- Starchy vegetables, legumes, and white carbohydrates: ½ cup equals 100 calories.
- Protein: One deck of cards equals 150 calories.
- One slice of bread equals 100 calories.
- One 12 oz. glass of beer equals 150 calories.
- One 5 oz. glass of wine equals 120 calories.
- Add the fat you used to cook the vegetables and protein—one tablespoon of any fat equals 100 calories.

Before you know it, your meal is 800 calories…and not because of the vegetables!

Rationale and benefits of this experiment:
Yet another way to be in control of your environment. If you estimate the calories in front of you, or if you read them on the menu, it will change your behavior. If there is too much on your plate, put half or one third aside for the next day. Or make better choices.

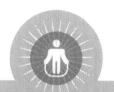

ACTIVITY LEVEL AND ENERGY

Experiment #65 – Describe How You Feel after Exercising

How is exercise treating you? We usually go to the gym with more or less enthusiasm. Some people know they really need it and enjoy the experience. Most of us go on a mission because we know we must for our health. We need many "Positive Automatic Thoughts" to motivate us. We need tricks, like having a gym bag in the car ready to go, or a buddy who will push us to go. We may not have yet found what we really like.

By Week 10 we are at Master Level and should have a pretty good idea of how we feel after exercising. I am not talking about the possible painful aftermath, but about how we feel in our heads. Are we quicker now at walking? Do we get out of the car more easily?

What is your level of energy, how do you sleep, how much longer can you work out? Is your concentration improving? Today think and write an essay about how you FEEL after you exercise, right after, but also in general.

I feel _____

_____

Rationale and benefits of this experiment:
By writing how you feel, and it is positive, you reinforce the pleasure pathway associated with exercise and activity in your brain.

EMOTIONS

Experiment #66 – Explore Boredom

Very often we experience boredom, which I said earlier is not an emotion. It is a temporary emptiness of the brain we should welcome. I do like these moments of stillness because I am never bored!

A "boredom window" allows for meditation, having a nice cup of tea, reading a book, coloring, knitting, going for a walk, or calling a friend.

Why is it then, that in these moments of boredom we open the fridge or rummage the shelves in search for cookies? It is because we live in such a fast-paced world we don't know how to deal with silence. We must be constantly occupied.

Having hobbies and projects helps. Next time you head to the fridge think about what led you there. Is food going to answer anything?

Next time you have a boredom episode, explore it. Be in the moment. Be seated somewhere comfortable and reflect on that silence. You should cherish it. It is not a hole in your soul. It is a moment of calm in your brain!

Rationale and benefits of this experiment:
You must learn to appreciate stillness and calm. Use these moments to give a break to your brain. The "going for food" is just an attempt to answer a void in your brain and fill it with mastication. Fill it with something more spiritual or creative.

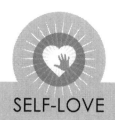

SELF-LOVE

Experiment #67 – Boost Your Motivation

By now you may have lost nine to 18 or more pounds. By the way, even if you "only" lost four pounds, it is a victory.

Get the equivalent of what you lost in something you can weigh in your kitchen (do you have a 10-pound bag of rice, I doubt it). You can also use weights you may have at home. Or you can do this experiment at the gym if they have stairs, or even better, a stair master.

Go up the stairs as usual. Then go up the stairs with the added weight representing what you have lost. Go up the stairs several times as if it is a workout. You will feel the difference with and without the extra weight you lost.

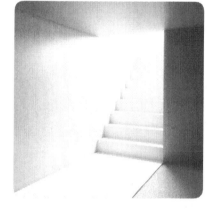

I make clients do this at my office and it is always such an eye opener. People are so proud. Focus on your heart beat, your breathing and how it changes with an extra load of weight.

Rationale and benefits of this experiment:
This experiment will reinforce your sense of success, and accomplishment, and will educate you on the importance of losing weight. This is a way to demonstrate physical benefits other than on a scale or looking in a mirror.

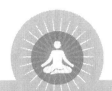

MINDFULNESS AND ZEN LIFE

Experiment #68 – Visualize the Energy in Foods

I call this the "Alive Factor" experiment. A food that is alive means it will bring you natural minerals, vitamins, anti-oxidants, and nutrients. It is optimal. The fresher, the more organic, and the simpler, the better it is for your health.

The energy of the earth is penetrating your body and nourishing every cell within your body. This carrot was planted and has grown thanks to water, sun, earth, and some love.

A cow fed naturally, happily in a pasture, and treated with respect will produce better milk and meat. A processed potato or stuff-based chips or protein bars are just an assembly of parts that were not supposed to be together but were glued.

Become good at giving foods an "Alive Factor" rating. The best foods will earn a 10. The most processed foods will get a zero. How are you eating? Visualize how this food is being processed in your body. Do you think we were supposed to eat preservatives, colorants, and emulsifiers? Do you believe it is optimal to eat processed hydrogenated fats and sugar laden ham or frozen dinners (yes, sugar is added there, too)?

Rationale and benefits of this experiment:
The purpose of this experiment is to get you closer to nature and natural foods. Eat a fresh local tomato in season and then have ketchup. Then, after reading the ketchup label, imagine what is happening in your body.

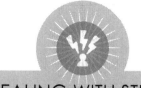

DEALING WITH STRESS

Experiment #69 – Learn to Be a Kid Again

We are so serious and so busy about our lives. We run from one activity to the other, rarely taking a break. I hope you have learned to take mini breaks by now. What I am trying to say is that we do not allow ourselves to be silly anymore. We are playful creatures. We like to have fun. We are engineered to laugh, smile, and be happy.

This week I am asking you to let your inner child get out of his shell. Do one thing to be silly. I remember one autumn season with my kids when they were younger. In Princeton there were mountains of leaves in the streets ready to be picked up. I stopped the car and we jumped on a pile. They could not believe their mother had done that. They still talk about it to this day.

Take the day and regularly measure the level of stress you feel. Notice the patterns, the way you feel, and the culprits. You can compare days of the week. Do this a few days this week.

Do ONE childish thing this week. Enjoy it, share the experience with friends or family or even colleagues.

Rationale and benefits of this experiment:
Being a child again brings you back to being able to be silly and doing things that are supposedly not appropriate for adults. But who said so? Multiply your happiness factor. Have fun. We only live once.

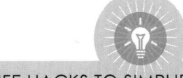

LIFE HACKS TO SIMPLIFY YOUR LIFE

Experiment #70 – Eliminate the Real Saboteurs

It is not easy to deal with saboteurs when they are
loved ones. You live with them, and they may
have a different lifestyle or eating
habits. This includes the partner who
comes home with a pint of chocolate ice cream
or pastry because he or she feels like having it.

You can learn to deal with saboteurs in Chapter 7
"I Deal with Saboteurs and Eat Mindfully"
in my book *Weight Loss Starts in Your Brain*.
However, we need to be firmer with the real
saboteurs, the ones who literally push us to eat or drink.

They push you because it reinforces THEIR behaviors. There
are also some dark reasons behind these pushing behaviors. The
pushers subconsciously don't want you to succeed. Not kidding.
Even very good friends.

You need to do three things:
1. Clarify once and for all that you will not go to these restaurants
   or eat this anymore. Make it clear they cannot push you.
   Say it nicely, like you learned in **Experiment #38**, where you
   expressed your WANTS.
2. If they don't get the message and you are on this new health
   quest, maybe it is time to see other people or avoid seeing
   these people as often.
3. Ignore their remarks or the push with a smile. Say "I am not
   interested." I guarantee after a while they will stop (or won't
   see you anymore).

Write down the list of your saboteurs and address the issues and how you will handle them.

Saboteur #1 _____

_____

_____

_____

Saboteur #2 _____

_____

_____

_____

Deal with only one person at a time. Prepare your speech or behavior. You are in charge. It is your body, your health, your mouth, and your choice. Nobody can tell you what to put in your mouth.

Rationale and benefits of this experiment:
You need to be in charge of your environment. You have cleaned your pantry, your wardrobe, and your office space, etc. You are eliminating negative energy. Saboteurs must be dealt with too, because as humans they can bully you into behaviors you don't want anymore.

Week 11

Who did you label as a "food saboteur?" Did you find a way to see them less or create neutral grounds?

How do you feel after exercising, hopefully like a million bucks? Describe this feeling in one word:

I feel _____

Are you getting better at assessing what is on your plate? What about this meal? **Estimate the calories:**

- 3 oz. salmon
- 2 cups salad with cut vegetables and vinaigrette
- ½ cup potatoes
- One 5 oz. glass of wine

My guess is that's _____ calories.

Answer: 500-600 calories

Now estimate this one:
A single patty beef hamburger with cheese, a bun, mayonnaise, ketchup, and a small portion of fries.

That sounds like _____ calories.

800-1,000 calories and zero vegetables

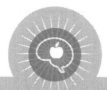

NUTRITION IQ AND FOOD EXPERIENCES

Experiment #71 – Be a Label Sleuth

Become an expert and be very curious about what is written on packaged foods.

Next time you go to a grocery shop, or while you are cleaning your pantry, look at the labels.

- How many servings are really in this bag of chips? Oh, I ate in fact 100 calories X three servings = 300 calories and not just 100 calories!
- How many grams of net carbohydrates (it will all become sugar in my blood) are in this bag? Remember net carbohydrates are total carbohydrates minus fiber.
- Look at the list of ingredients. What type of sugar did they add?
- And what about preservatives, colorants, emulsifiers, and thickeners?
- Did they use real potatoes to make these chips, or is this an amalgamation of potato puree and corn starches?
- Is this real pure peanut butter? Sometimes they add protein powder and extra fat, usually palm oil.
- Is this pure honey or did they add glucose?

Rationale and benefits of this experiment:
The more curious and informed you are, the better choices you will make. By just systematically looking at labels, it gives you pause, and takes away the impulse of opening the bag without mindfulness. It will change your behaviors, I can guarantee it.

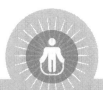

ACTIVITY LEVEL AND ENERGY

Experiment #72 – Become More Active in General

You upped the exercise factor and are walking longer or faster. I want to speak about the multiple ways you can burn more calories during the day outside of exercising. It has been proven a highly active lifestyle is more desirable than one hour of exercise a day.

- Are you walking as much as you should (10,000 steps a day)?
- Are you taking the stairs versus the elevator?
- Are you parking your car far away from the shopping center?
- Are you being active in your garden? Or are you doing handy work in the house?
- Do you have a walking or standing desk at the office or at home?
- Do you take regular breaks when in front of your computer (some smart step counters can alert you to move)?
- Do you squat or lunge spontaneously during the day?

Rationale and benefits of this experiment:
Being more active throughout the will boost your metabolism and force you to burn calories non-stop. It can help you burn an extra 500-1,000 calories a day without going to the gym! This does not give you permission to skip the gym however! You still need strength and cardio training.

EMOTIONS

Experiment #73 – Count to 10

You tried the "snap out of it method" in **Experiment #52**, but when dealing with an emotion, it sometimes works better if you face the fact that you want a treat. Just before you reach out to the snack, slowly count to 10. Remember to breathe mindfully as we did in **Experiment #20** in Week 3.

1...2...3...4...5...6...7...8...9...10

Counting slowly to 10 is a way to slow down your impulse, calm your brain, and give yourself enough time to choose an alternative action:

- Walk away from the temptation or throw it in the garbage can (I have done that).
- Imagine what this temptation will not solve.
- Think about your vision board and past victories.
- Evaluate the lack of nutritional value of that food (remember **Experiment #33** and the three questions).
- Recite your mantra etc.

This is not the distraction method from **Experiment #56** which allows you to put your brain on another bandwidth. This is just a counting game. You are facing your temptation.

Rationale and benefits of this experiment:
This a battle with your willpower. You are fighting the temptation with mindfulness or facts and information. It must be done. We must learn to stand in front of these foods and resist because they are constantly around us.

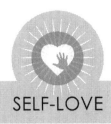

SELF-LOVE

Experiment #74 – Imagine You Are a Rose

Be creative, be artistic. Art is underappreciated as a tool to deal with emotions. Imagine yourself as a rose, or another flower.

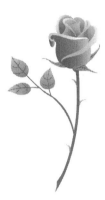

Every time you breathe in, the petals close, and every time you breathe out, the petals open, caressed by the sun and the wind. The rose offers its beautiful glory to the universe. This rose is magnificent. It is you.

Each time you exhale, expel a negative emotion or thought about yourself. It could be "I am not beautiful enough," or "I am a failure." Imagine the negative thoughts flowing out and disappearing in the wind.

You feel lighter. You are letting go. It comes from deep inside. It is gone, and you can close the flower again. As you close the flower, imagine a positive thought or emotion to replace the negativity, that makes you feel vibrant and happy. Remember all the things you love about yourself! You could say as you inhale: "I am becoming a new me," "I am more confident," or "I am happier."

You can repeat the experiment, focusing on one specific negative thought at a time. As you do this you become lighter and freer. You will feel as beautiful as the rose.

Rationale and benefits of this experiment:
This is one more way to help you focus on what is positive and beautiful about yourself.

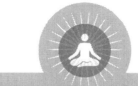

MINDFULNESS AND ZEN LIFE

Experiment #75 – Treat vs. Trigger

There are foods that will trigger a want for more. They will launch you into a vicious circle of never ending cravings. We are talking about sugar.

Let's consider an alternative. Maybe there is a TREAT that will make you happy but will not launch you on a wild sugar journey.

I have an example to share. I love chocolate. If I have 65% cacao chocolate, I will eat the whole bar. If I have the 85 or 90% chocolate, which is much lower in sugar and higher in fat, I am content with one or two squares. Another trigger for me is coffee. I always want a sweet with it, like a cookie. Why cookie, because coffee also increases your blood sugar, even black coffee.

Enter your triggers and try to replace them with a treat. Treats are usually higher quality products with real ingredients. Do the experiment.

TRIGGERS	TREATS

Rationale and benefits of this experiment:
The more you know how your body reacts to certain foods, the more you can make better choices, without always feeling deprived.

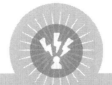

DEALING WITH STRESS

Experiment #76 – Learn to Say No!

Next time you are experiencing a stressful situation, which is often triggered by others, learn to get out of it. Why suffer the stress of something you did not want, you never asked for, and you were not consulted about?

Remember the dinner your partner organized during a busy week without telling you? You were told the day before. You were asked to bake a dessert, on your way back from the airport. You did not enjoy that party, you were too tired.

Next time something like this occurs, even if it is at the last minute, ask yourself these three questions:

1. What is in it for me? Is it worth the extra stress?
2. Will people hate me forever if I say no?
3. Can it be postponed?

I am not telling you to become a party pooper. But after you answer these three questions, decide what your position is and how you will communicate it.

Rationale and benefits of this experiment:
Very often we let people we love, and those we don't love, decide and manage our lives without ever asking or considering what we want or need at that point. Be in charge of your life and it will be much less stressful. Saying NO is very powerful and allows for a more focused life.

LIFE HACKS TO SIMPLIFY YOUR LIFE

Experiment #77 – Is Your Budget Aligned with Your Goals?

Have a look at your monthly budget and organize it as such:

	$	%
Housing		
Food		
Cars		
Clothes and Grooming (hairdresser, etc.)		
Education for Children		
Education (new diploma, classes, etc.)		
Savings in General		
Vacation (savings)		
Leisure (restaurants, movies, etc.)		
Health (insurance, doctors, medications, supplements)		
Other (garden, home improvement, gifts, etc.)		
Exercise, Relaxation, Gym Fees, New Equipment, etc.		

How much and what percent is spent in each bucket? How much is spent on getting healthy? How much on medications to combat side effects of not exercising, eating not so well, and being sedentary? Note how long it took.

Rationale and benefits of this experiment:
Let us examine how we spend our money. Does the budget support our health goals? Can we substitute splurging on expensive snacks with paying for a personal trainer?

Week 12

The final week!

The celebration. The results. The joy and the changes that occurred. Please get ready to finish with panache!

At the end of the week, take pictures and enter your data.

WEEK 1								
WEEK 2								
WEEK 3								
WEEK 4								
WEEK 5								
WEEK 6								
WEEK 7								
WEEK 8								
WEEK 9								
WEEK 10								
WEEK 11								
WEEK 12								

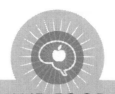

NUTRITION IQ AND FOOD EXPERIENCES

Experiment #78 – What if I Have a Snack Attack?

Let's be practical. You can experience a snack attack. Your energy may go down especially in the afternoon. It is important to be prepared so you do not venture into dangerous office kitchens, meeting rooms, and vending machines with unhealthy snacks.

Veronique, you just asked us to stop snacking. Yes, ideally, we should not be snacking if we are not hungry. But sometimes we are hungry or in need of an energy boost.

Keep healthy snacks in your purse, car, or office. I suggest protein-based snacks. They are better at calming hunger than carbohydrate-rich snacks that will launch you on a blood glucose level roller coaster (Read the chapter on sugar in *Weight Loss Starts in Your Brain*). Good choices are:

- Nuts in a reasonable quantity (no more than 10-15 nuts).
- Meat-based snacks.
- A high protein content bar (20g minimum) with no more than 15-20g of net carbohydrates. Limit to 150 calories total.
- Make sure there is some good fat as well, as fat will also make you feel more satiated (like a piece of avocado or nut butters).

Rationale and benefits of this experiment:
This will help you be READY and avoid the sugar craving vicious circle. Observe what happens. Did you really need that snack?

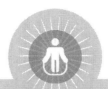

ACTIVITY LEVEL AND ENERGY

Experiment #79 – The Multiple Health Benefits of Exercising

In Week 9 **Experiment #58**, we asked you to notice how your body changed. We asked you to examine how you felt after exercising in **Experiment #65**.

As we enter the final days in this book, I would like you to remind yourself of ALL the benefits of exercising. Exercise is proven to positively impact memory, sleep, stress relief, stamina, focus, brain performance, and aging, etc.

Write down the benefits exercising or simply being more active has on your body and mind. It can be very personal. One day a grandmother told me that since she did The CogniDiet® Program and started to exercise again, she could play with her grandchildren. Another woman told me she could run with her husband again.

Here are my benefits from exercising: _____

_____

_____

_____

Rationale and benefits of this experiment:
This essay will solidify the value of your increased exercise regimen from a holistic point of view.
Keep this in mind when you go to the gym tired and unmotivated. You are in it for the long-term benefits.

EMOTIONS

Experiment #80 – Why Eating Is Not the Answer

Now that we are at the end of the program, we need to switch gears to the long term.

What have you discovered about your emotions and how they trigger food cravings? Have you been able to tackle some of them? Did you find ways to cope with them better, even get to the bottom of some?

I am asking you in this final experiment to write a letter about why eating is not the answer when an emotion, pleasant or unpleasant, hits you.

Eating is not the answer when I am sad because ... Or eating is not the answer when I am angry because ...

It is up to you, write this essay and read it often. Remember your needs and wants. Remember how you feel after the binge. Remember how you feel during the emotion.

Rationale and benefits of this experiment:
This essay will put on paper the feelings and deep emotions that hit you before the chocolate or the candy hunt. This will help you express all the reasons that food is not the answer. I highly recommend at the end of this essay that you write an action plan. The answer may be to avoid some people and situations, or that you may need some psychotherapy. Or simply just snap out of it!

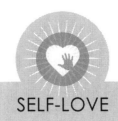

SELF-LOVE

Experiment #81 – A Love Letter to Myself

Take a pen and write yourself a letter about everything you learned about yourself, your transformation, and your level of happiness after these 12 weeks.

This is an experiment you could do after each week.

You had to do a lot. Some of you may have abandoned ship, gotten discouraged, or became bored. If so, I advise you go back to square one and re-do the 12 weeks at a slower pace.

Handwrite this letter and once written, keep it with you and read it every day. Perhaps add a before and after picture to the letter. And every day when you read the letter, compliment yourself. You will feel as beautiful as the rose.

Rationale and benefits of this experiment:
I don't think I have to explain this anymore. You've got the spirit. Be bold. This is not a time to be humble or shy. Just own your transformation.

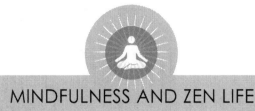

MINDFULNESS AND ZEN LIFE

Experiment #82 – The Blindfold Dinner

This is a fun experiment. You need somebody to cook for you if you want the extra pleasure of discovering what you are eating. If not, simply put on a sleeping mask before someone serves your plate. You cannot see what is put on your plate!

The idea is also to eat in silence and be focused on the food. Be very mindful, chew as recommended, place your silverware on the table after each morsel. You will be slowed down because you have to struggle to find the food on your plate. This is why, because I have done this multiple times, I recommend you cook something easy to slice, such as sausages or well-cooked vegetables.

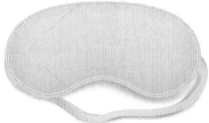

When you feel you are no longer hungry, stop eating. Take off your mask off and gauge what portion you ate. It is extra fun if guess what you ate, and what spices and herbs were used.

I will not share the rationale for this experiment
because I would be exposing its purpose and influence you. But I bet you will have many interesting findings and "a-ha" moments. Enjoy!

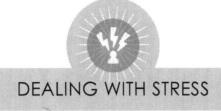

DEALING WITH STRESS

Experiment #83 – Write a Plan to Change Your Life

In this program, we helped you discover the sources of your stress and then taught you to cope with them. We also tried to help you eliminate short term stress.

But often the biggest source of stress is a responsibility you cannot escape. A job you cannot leave, a commute you cannot stop, a marriage you cannot get out of. A life that binds you to an inevitable frustrating litany of chores and events you do not want.

You may have a rather high level of Zen factor, you may be a saint, or a victim.

As you know, stress is taking a toll on your health. Stress is devouring your soul and robbing you of your most cherished dreams.

I say it often to some of my clients. If you do not manage or eliminate sources of stress, they will never disappear.

They impact your life. They destroy your health. In this final week I am asking you to at least start to draft a long-term plan of what needs to change in your life.

Write what you want to eliminate on the next page, and then determine the steps you must take.

My Life-Changing Plan

_____

_____

_____

_____

_____

_____

_____

_____

_____

_____

_____

_____

_____

_____

_____

Rationale and benefits of this experiment:
If something has to really change, you need to start making the change happen for you to live your life to the fullest.

LIFE HACKS TO SIMPLIFY YOUR LIFE

Experiment #84 – Rate Yourself and Go Back to Square One

Based on all the previous experiments in Life Hacks we asked you to perform, you must have noticed we kept asking you to simplify and eliminate what is in the way of you living your healthy life.

We are always surprised to see how a day is organized, and then a week, because we follow a flow rather than being more assertive about what we want and need.

I am a big believer, and this is the last experiment, that if we do not stand up for what we want, nobody else will. And I know putting ourselves first is not always easy, especially for women. If we want to live in harmony, we must do it as much as we can.

On a scale from zero to 10, how good do you think you were at cutting the dead branches, and clearing the path for your healthy life? Did you do the experiments? That in itself requires time and dedication. If you score a zero, maybe you should consider thinking hard about doing this program again.

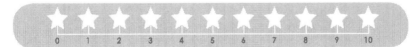

Rationale and benefits of this experiment:
Please take the time to take care of yourself. But also, be honest with yourself. We cannot have everything. We must choose what matters most.

Yes, You Have Graduated!

You are a Master!

You are in charge of your life and your environment.

You decide what and when to do something that is good, or not so good for you.

You have discovered so many new things about yourself.

You may be 33 pounds, or more, lighter, like one of the participants in my clinical trial. She has now lost 80 pounds and has maintained this weight for over two years.

Celebrate by treating yourself with something very nice and special that will last and be a reminder of your many victories. Be proud.

I lost _____ pounds

I feel _____

Made in the USA
San Bernardino, CA
15 March 2019